WKH-0003

Implementing Early Intervention in Psychosis

A Guide to Establishing Early Psychosis Services

JANE EDWARDS BA (HONS), MA (CLIN PSYCH)
PHD, MAPS
Deputy Clinical Director
Early Psychosis Prevention and Intervention
Centre (EPPIC)/Mental Health Services for
Kids and Youths (MH-SKY), and Fellow of the
Departments of Psychiatry and Psychology
University of Melbourne, Parkville, Australia

PATRICK D MCGORRY MBBS, PHD, FRANZCP
Professor and Director, Early Psychosis Prevention
and Intervention Centre (EPPIC)/Mental Health Services
for Kids and Youth (MH-SKY), and Department of
Psychiatry, University of Melbourne, Parkville, Australia

MARTIN DUNITZ

© 2002 Martin Dunitz Ltd, a member of the Taylor & Francis group

First published in the United Kingdom in 2002 by Martin Dunitz Ltd, The Livery House, 7–9 Pratt Street, London NW1 0AE

Tel: +44 (0) 20 7482 2202
Fax: +44 (0) 20 7267 0159
E-mail: info@dunitz.co.uk
Website: http://www.dunitz.co.uk

Reprinted 2002

A CIP record for this book is available from the British Library.

ISBN 1 84184 053 X

Although every effort has been made to ensure that all owners of copyright material have been acknowledged in this publication, we would be glad to acknowledge in subsequent reprints or editions any omissions brought to our attention.

Distributed in the USA by
Fulfilment Center
Taylor & Francis
7625 Empire Drive
Florence, KY 41042, USA
Toll Free Tel.: +1 800 634 7064
E-mail: cserve@routledge_ny.com

Distributed in Canada by
Taylor & Francis
74 Rolark Drive
Scarborough, Ontario M1R 4G2, Canada
Toll Free Tel.: +1 877 226 2237
E-mail: tal_fran@istar.ca

Distributed in the rest of the world by
TPS Limited
Cheriton House
North Way
Andover, Hampshire SP10 5BE, UK
Tel.: +44 (0)1264 332424
E-mail: salesorder.tandf@thomsonpublishingservices.co.uk

Composition by Wearset Ltd, Boldon, Tyne and Wear
Printed and bound in Great Britain by The Cromwell Press, Trowbridge

Contents

Foreword

'The longest journey begins with a single step'

Advances in medicine and public health generally derive from some scientific discovery or breakthrough (for example, the discovery of antibiotics, vaccines for prevention of infectious disease, insulin for the treatment of diabetes, radiation and chemotherapy for cancer and the isolation of the human immunoinsuffiency virus [HIV] at which protease inhibitors are targeted). However, advances of equal import have been achieved through the recognition of how the application of existing knowledge in new health care services and procedures can have profound therapeutic impact; to wit the enormous benefits of the invention of sterile techniques including simple handwashing, universal prenatal care delivery, the codification of procedures for cardiopulmonary resuscitation. Although the care of patients with mental illnesses has benefited greatly from numerous discoveries (both serendipitous and rationalized) of psychotropic drugs, momentous innovations of services and procedures have been rare. In this context, the significance of the information embodied in this book and the milestone of its publication can be most appropriately viewed and fully appreciated. In doing so one can only arrive at the conclusion that this volume is a seminal work, which will have broad and enduring effects on public mental health and service delivery systems.

Whether the origins of the early psychosis concept and research focus began in the 1980s with the work of Crow,

Johnstone, Kane and Lieberman, or in the earlier landmark studies of Beiser and May, or were prefigured in the catamnestic studies of Bleuler (M), Ciompi and Huber, or were implicit in the concept of progression and deterioration that was fundamental to Kraepelin's original description of dementia praecox, there can be no doubt that the model for early identification and intervention, which is the subject of this book, represents its culmination. The pioneering efforts of McGorry, Edwards and their colleagues have served to unify the relevant scientific research, service delivery systems and mental health policy in a way that has alleviated the usual 'bottleneck' of delays that routinely impedes the translation of scientific research into clinical practice. Indeed their efforts have mobilized and inspired not just a research field, but a veritable movement with an official organization (International Early Psychosis Association) and manifesto (see Chapter 9) which has at times engendered excitement of evangelical proportions. But at the heart of this enterprise, stripped of all the political and ideological trappings, are a conceptual model, organizational plan and body of experience that is ready for prime time. Hence the purpose of this book is to provide a 'guide to establishing early psychosis services'.

It is exciting to envision the ramifications of such early psychosis services. They will require the establishment of new clinical service infrastructures, new training models for mental health care clinicians and, most importantly, provide earlier and better treatment for patients with psychotic disorders that will almost certainly result in decreased morbidity from their illnesses and vastly better outcomes than such patients have historically had. This will truly constitute a major advance in mental health care for which our colleagues from 'down under' deserve recognition and credit.

Jeffrey A Lieberman MD
University of North Carolina School of Medicine
Chapel Hill, North Carolina, USA

Preface

"The best progressive ideas are those that include a strong enough dose of provocation to make its supporters feel proud of being original, but at the same time attract so many adherents that the risk of being an isolated exception is immediately averted by the noisy approval of a triumphant crowd." Kundera (1996, p. 273)

The recognition and management of early psychosis has become a popular focus among clinicians, researchers and service reformers in recent years. Despite the pessimism shrouding schizophrenia, which remains to be definitively dispelled by more dramatic therapeutic advances, the creation of the first episode research focus in the early 1980s by Crow and colleagues in the UK, and Kane and colleagues in the USA resulted in a solid foundation for a more optimistic stance in treating schizophrenia and related psychoses. We began our research endeavours in schizophrenia around the same time with an exclusive focus on first episode cases. This immediately highlighted how difficult and arbitrary it was to access timely intervention; how crude and limited our approach really was, and how much iatrogenic damage was being inflicted on vulnerable patients and families. Since then substantial research has been undertaken which has converged in support of the early intervention paradigm. Some researchers have remained sceptical about the potential value of earlier detection and an enhanced early treatment approach, insisting on a definitive evidence base before any reforms are engineered. Other researchers and most clinicians, patients and families believe that staged reform in practice and service provision is necessary to enable further evidence to be collected. In any case, to argue against early detection and optimal treatment seems to defend the indefensible, namely to require patients and families to reach a high threshold of risk, disruption, or deterioration to access acute care and demonstrate a relapsing or chronically disabled pattern to justify continuing care. This is a classic state of closing the stable door after the horse has bolted. It reinforces the pessimistic stereotype of schizophrenia and is a residual consequence of the asylum model which persists in the era of community psychiatry.

This book is intended to be part of the reform process by which this model of care is transcended and all the benefits of existing and emerging knowledge deployed during the phase of illness in which they are most likely to be of benefit in minimising the potentially disastrous, even fatal, effects of psychotic disorder. Psychiatric service reform is a sociological and political process informed by scientific evidence. We respect the fundamental importance of evidence as a

guide and safeguard in reform; however, it is naive to rely on evidence alone to bring about change just as evidence of this type is not the only legitimate influence on the direction and pace of reform.

Chapter 1 provides an introduction to the rationale for early intervention and introduces the treatment approach. Chapters 2–4 draw on the 10-module *Early Psychosis Training Pack* (McGorry and Edwards, 1997) and on McGorry and Jackson (1999), and provides an updated brief overview of phase specific service elements central to early detection and intervention service development efforts. Descriptions of components from the Early Psychosis Prevention and Intervention Centre (EPPIC), Melbourne, Australia, are used throughout Chapters 2–4 to illustrate service applications. The aim is to draw on our service delivery experience to inform the reader about the scope of possible specialised interventions in early psychosis. Clearly other services will have their own possibilities – the EPPIC components and practical resources for clinicians are described with the intention of providing short cuts for those evolving new and more refined approaches – a 'biblio proxy' for an EPPIC site visit. Chapter 4 contains more numerous examples of the EPPIC service elements, reflecting the substantial efforts that have gone into developing 'tools for the toolkit' of the early psychosis clinician.

The EPPIC model is described in Chapter 5 (i.e. how the elements fit together), and comprehensive systems of care for early psychosis, two in operation in Europe and two in Canada, are outlined in some detail. The purpose here is for the reader to appreciate the developmental trajectory of these state of the art services and gain an understanding of how specialized interventions for early psychosis are delivered within a service context. The reader is advised to have an atlas handy and may need to seek additional information about health policy at the regional/national levels to fully appreciate service developments in context.

The second half of the book describes strategies to assist with early psychosis service development – putting the foci into practice (a phase which may last 2–3 years) and making the transition to an enduring system. Many of the points made in Chapters 6–8 are illustrated by examples of early psychosis services occurring throughout the world. Chapter 6 outlines a 9-step model to getting started. Chapter 7 concerns the comprehensive evaluation of an early psychosis service, vital to programme survival and essential to expansion of the knowledge base. Chapter 8 deals with elements of 'becoming real' (Rosen et al, 1997) such as

specialist versus generalist model considerations and staff training. The book concludes with Chapter 9, advancing a consensus statement to be presented in its final form at the Third International Conference on Early Psychosis to be held in 2002 – a contribution to the sound ethical base required to progress the field on multiple fronts. It would be fair to say that in some instances these draft guidelines are more specific than our own position provided in earlier chapters – Chapter 9 reflects a broader viewpoint which has, at times, extended our thinking.

Two caveats are required. First, there has been a massive boom in service development and the examples provided here are by no means exhaustive. Readers may be well aware of early psychosis services not mentioned in the text and, hopefully, many more programmes that are in progress will emerge shortly. Second, the pocketbook aims to target a wide audience. For some the text may appear too simple, for others it will be too complex. The guide is intended to be used as a source – the references, web sites and e-mail contacts provide important information.

Acknowledgements

We would like to acknowledge EPPIC staff and patients who have contributed to the body of knowledge summarized in this book. Many correspondents generously drafted or edited sections describing their own services and the collegiate atmosphere in which this occurred has been inspiring. The diligent support of Sue Leitinger throughout the project, particularly with regard to the tracking of both resources and reviewers, is much appreciated. Bernie Cram designed the cover, patiently encouraging us to transcend 'funky'. Tony James cheerfully assisted with the editing process during the final stages and we appreciate his skilled involvement. We are grateful to the 26 international consultants for constructive feedback on the draft consensus statement, now revised and contained in Chapter 9. We also wish to thank Jean Addington, Jan Olav Johannessen, Thomas McGlashan and Ashok Malla for taking the time to read the entire manuscript and for their helpful and encouraging comments. Our long associations with trusted and respected early psychosis friends and colleagues has made the endeavour even more rewarding. We look forward to further progress in the field of early psychosis with the hope that this will translate into benefits for young people and their families at all phases of illness.

Correspondents

D Addington
J Addington
D Albiston
GP Amminger
C Aragona
D Bathgate
J Beckman
R Bell
C Bensemann
G Berger
M Birchwood
J Bywaters
S Catts
E Chen
C Crotty
J Cullberg
K Crisp
L Drew
R Duff
J Duval
T Ehman
K Elkins
C Gardiner
G Garland
J Gleeson
J Gorrell
S Haines
M Hambrecht
L Hanson
M Harris
L Henry
A Herman
H Hobbs

D Howe
C Jackson
H Jackson
JO Johannessen
H Krstev
TK Larsen
I Law
S Lewis
E Lines
B MacEwan
A Malla
R May
E McDonald
T McGlashan
W McFarlane
I Melle
T Miller
B Moss
S Nightingale
S Noseworthy
K Paterson
K Pennell
L Phillips
N Preston
P Power
F Resch
T Sale
K Savicki
S Shah
W Smith
S Spurr
M Still
K Tee
E Temple

D Wade
J Walters
B Wentzell
D Whitehorn
L Wong
AM Wright
R Zipursky

International Consultants – Chapter 9
J Addington (Canada)
GP Amminger (Austria)
A Barbato (Italy)
S Catts (Australia)
E Chen (Hong Kong)
S Chhim (Cambodia)
SA Chong (Singapore)
J Cullberg (Sweden)
L Grosso (France)
M Louzã (Brazil)
M Hambrecht (Germany)

M Keshavan (USA)
JO Johannessen (Norway)
DL Johnson (USA)
S Lewis (UK)
J Lieberman (USA)
B MacEwan (Canada)
A Malla (Canada)
R May (UK)
T McGlashan (USA)
MG Merlo (Switzerland)
M Nordentoft (Denmark)
S Nightingale (New Zealand)
D Perkins (USA)
R Thara (India)
K Yamamoto (Japan)

Jane Edwards and Patrick D McGorry
Melbourne, Australia,
February 2002

Dedication

In memory of Carlo Perris (1928–2000)

Early intervention in psychosis – rationale and overview of clinical management

During the 1990s there was growing optimism about the prospects for better outcomes in schizophrenia and related psychoses. Clinicians and policy makers were enthusiastic about the reform needed to achieve this goal because of the sound logic behind it, the poor access and quality of care previously available to young people with early psychosis, and the increasing evidence that better outcomes can be achieved.

Some of this optimism flowed from the development of a new generation of antipsychotic medications that had greater efficacy and fewer side effects. A second factor was the belated recognition that a special focus on the early phases of psychotic illness could result in a substantial reduction in morbidity and in a better quality of life for patients and their families. This is not a new idea, having been formulated in the 19th century, further developed during the pre-antipsychotic era by Sullivan (1927) and subsequently by others (Cameron 1938, Meares 1959). However, the concept of early intervention remained dormant for decades until the publication of some key research studies (e.g. Falloon 1992, Loebel et al 1992, McGlashan 1996, McGorry 1998) and a rapid growth of enthusiasm during the 1990s.

The research revealed the special needs of young people

with early psychosis, the iatrogenic effects of standard care and the potential for a range of secondary prevention opportunities. Key failures in care included:

- prolonged delays in accessing effective treatment, which usually occurs in the context of a severe behavioural crisis
- crude, often traumatic and alienating initial treatment strategies
- poor continuity of care
- poor engagement of the patient in treatment

Usually, young people do not gain access to care until they demonstrate severe risk to themselves or others, or develop a relapsing and chronically disabling pattern of illness that requires ongoing care.

The innovative work of Falloon (1992), the increasing devolution of mental health care into community settings, and a renaissance in biological and psychological treatments for psychosis have added to the momentum for early intervention. Growth of neuroscientific research in schizophrenia has injected further optimism. Several countries have developed national mental health strategies or frameworks to guide major reform in mental health care and encourage a preventive approach. A large number of groups around the world have now established clinical programmes and research focusing on early psychosis. This blend of science and

social movement has the potential to lead to a substantial change in the way these illnesses are managed.

Rationale for early intervention
Primary prevention of schizophrenia and related disorders remains out of reach, but there are excellent prospects for early intervention and secondary prevention. The latter can lead to:

- early detection of new cases
- shortening the delays to effective treatment
- provision of optimal and sustained treatment in the early 'critical period' of the first few years of illness

To reduce the impact and burden of psychotic disorders would be a major achievement. It may even be possible to reduce their prevalence, by delaying the onset of illness, reducing the time spent living with disability, or accelerating recovery.

The full promise of improved quality of care has not yet been realized despite the development of highly effective treatments (Hegarty et al 1994) because we have failed to translate these advances to the real world beyond the randomized controlled trial. Even with existing knowledge, substantial reductions in prevalence and improvements in quality of life are possible for patients, provided societies are prepared to pay for it.

Evidence is critical if there is to be a shift in attitudes and clinical practice, but how much evidence is required before a change in practice is warranted? We should remember that the alternative to early, optimal intervention is delayed and substandard treatment with all its consequences (Lieberman and Fenton 2000). Even in developed countries, the timing and quality of standard care is relatively poor. In developing countries, a significant proportion of cases never receives treatment (Padmavathi et al 1998). Evidence is needed, but there are also obvious clinical and common-sense drivers for more timely, widespread and better quality treatment.

Potential benefits of early intervention and treatment in psychotic illness

Early intervention may help prevent the often significant biological, social and psychological deterioration that can occur in the early years following onset of a psychotic disorder (Birchwood and Macmillan 1993). Significant delays before effective treatment is initiated, or secondary morbidity resulting from aspects of management, can hamper preventive efforts. Potential benefits of early intervention include:

- reduced morbidity
- more rapid recovery
- better prognosis
- preservation of psychosocial skills
- preservation of family and social supports
- decreased need for hospitalization.

Conceptual framework for early intervention

Mrazek and Haggerty (1994) developed a framework for conceptualizing, implementing and evaluating preventive interventions within the full spectrum of interventions for mental disorders (Figure 1.1). They classified preventive interventions as universal, selective or indicated. *Universal* preventive interventions are focused on the whole population (e.g. immunization and prevention of smoking), while *selective* preventive measures are aimed at asymptomatic subgroups of the population with a higher than average risk of becoming ill (e.g. annual mammograms for women with a positive

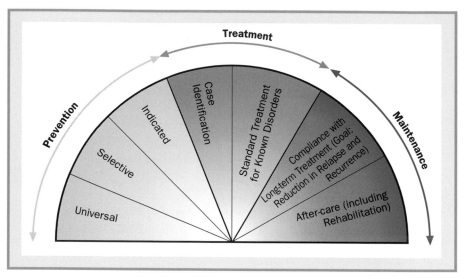

Figure 1.1
Spectrum of intervention in mental disorders.
Adapted with permission of National Academy Press, Washington, DC, from Mrazek PJ, Haggerty RJ, eds
(1994) Reducing Risks for Mental Disorders. *Washington, DC: National Academy Press.*

family history of breast cancer). *Indicated* prevention is targeted at individuals known to be at high risk of a specific disorder.

'Early intervention' in first-episode psychosis incorporates the concept of indicated prevention, which necessitates the identification of people with subthreshold symptoms that confer a high risk for a more severe disorder. This potentially constitutes a form of primary prevention. There are also two secondary foci:

- early case detection
- optimal management of the first episode of illness and the subsequent 'critical period'

Tertiary prevention involves reducing the long-term impact and burden of the disorder. In Figure 1.2 these different types of intervention are related to stages of illness.

Prepsychotic intervention
Background

Prepsychotic intervention is a form of indicated prevention. It has great potential but currently remains an issue for research rather than practice. Universal and selective approaches to prevention of psychotic illnesses are out of reach at present.

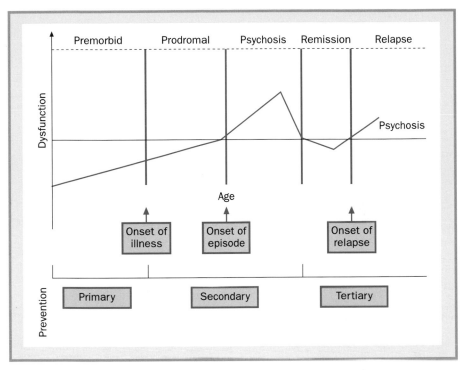

Figure 1.2
Stages of schizophrenia and prevention types.
Adapted with permission of Taylor & Francis from Johannessen JO, Larsen TK, McGlashan T (1999) Duration of untreated psychosis: an important target for intervention in schizophrenia? Nord J Psychiatry **53**:275–283.

The concept of prepsychotic intervention is controversial. In some cases the subthreshold clinical features will, in fact, be proved to have been 'prodromal' to a clearly defined psychotic illness. In other cases they will be 'false-positive' symptoms in people who do not develop a psychotic illness. Nevertheless, many people with subthreshold symptoms will need treatment for their disabling or distressing symptoms, regardless of the long-term outcome or diagnosis. Help-seeking and a need for treatment are not perfectly correlated with the threshold for a formal diagnosis (Frances 1998, Regier et al 1998, Spitzer 1998).

Clinicians have two options in responding to subthreshold symptoms. First, they can treat what is already present and, second, they can try to reduce the risk of the existing syndrome worsening or evolving into a more serious condition such as acute psychosis. The first option is not controversial and is good clinical care, but the benefit of the second approach remains unproven.

Symptoms experienced prior to a psychotic episode

Symptoms experienced prior to the onset of a clearly defined psychotic episode can include:

- changes in affect – suspiciousness, depression, anxiety, mood swings, feelings of tension, irritability, anger
- changes in cognition – odd ideas, vagueness, difficulties with concentration or recall
- changes in perception of self, of other people, of the world at large
- physical and perceptual changes – sleep disturbances, appetite changes, somatic complaints, loss of energy or motivation, perceptual disturbances

Prepsychotic intervention in the real world

Deficits in social functioning are primarily established during the prepsychotic or prodromal phase, when there is active illness but individuals have not yet passed a diagnostic threshold. The level of psychosocial development achieved by the end of the prodromal phase strongly influences the further social course of the disorder by setting a 'ceiling' for recovery (Häfner et al 1995, 1999).

Psychotic illnesses are rarely clinically active in childhood. Although an early vulnerability may exist in a proportion of cases, other environmental risk factors (Mahy et al 1999) and problems with adolescent brain development (Rapoport et al 1999) come into play during adolescence or later, usually months or years prior to the emergence of the defining features of psychotic disorder (McGorry et al, 2001a).

Recently it has become possible to identify people at very high risk of transition to psychosis through an approach termed the 'close-in' strategy (Bell 1992). Such young people are already distressed and functioning poorly, and are willing to accept professional help (see Chapter 2). Even with good psychosocial care, about 40% of patients at very high risk make the transition to first-episode psychosis within a 12-month follow-up period.

A range of ethical and conceptual issues needs to be considered in relation to this emerging field (see Chapter 8). However, the patients have significant disability and are seeking help. They must be distinguished from a subgroup of the general population who report isolated psychotic symptoms in the apparent absence of distress, disability or progressive change, and who do not desire assistance (Van Os et al 2000).

Further research is urgently required to clarify the treatments that will alleviate distress and disability and reduce the risk of subsequent psychosis. In the interim there is a need for a clinical response from psychiatrists, community mental health services and primary care, because these young people are highly symptomatic and at increased risk of suicide, substance misuse and vocational failure.

What should the clinician do when approached by a young person or by the family of a young person who appears to be at high risk? Some of the possible approaches are outlined later in this book (see Chapter 2), but in brief:

- If the symptoms are non-specific, especially if they are of recent onset and there is no family history of psychosis, then the approach should be general and supportive. This could include treating any specific features, such as depression, panic or obsessive–compulsive symptoms, with a psychosocial approach.
- Those meeting the criteria of very high risk can be offered initial psychosocial treatment, with or without syndrome-based drug treatments, aimed at the relief

of such distress and disability. What the patient and family should be told about the level of risk of future psychosis has been debated, but in our experience an open approach of disclosure, guided by the curiosity of the patient and family, has worked well.

- Not uncommonly, the parents of the young person will be concerned about vocational failure and social withdrawal in their child, but will be unable to persuade them to attend for assessment.
- If patients have problems relating to stigma and self-stigmatization, it is appropriate to find a way for the young person to be assessed and offered help in a nonstigmatizing manner. This can be accomplished through home visits by the family doctor, by the school counsellor, or by mobile mental health teams linked to youth health services or mental health services. Early intervention teams can be located in mainstream community facilities to facilitate such assessments and avoid stigma.

If psychosis does emerge and the symptoms cross the threshold for antipsychotic therapy, this focus on vulnerable, prepsychotic or potentially prodromal individuals will have already established a therapeutic relationship when the young person was less severely ill. This should facilitate acceptance of recommended medication and help avoid hospitalization. In addition, the duration of untreated psychosis is reduced to an absolute minimum.

Antipsychotic medications should generally be avoided in the prepsychotic phase. However, they could be considered in patients who meet the criteria for very high risk and who are rapidly deteriorating with increasing suicidality or risk of violence, or have increasingly disorganized, stigmatizing or embarrassing behaviours.

Early detection of first-episode psychosis

Background

Early case detection aimed at shortening delays in access to treatment should reduce the prevalence and morbidity of psychotic illnesses provided there is an effective form of treatment available. The average duration of untreated psychosis has been found to be between 1 and 2 years (Johannessen 2001). Delays in starting effective treatment may diminish their chances of complete recovery and/or slow the recovery process. Even if the response to treatment remains good after a significant delay, there is still a powerful human and medical argument for making effective treatment available to young people as early as possible in order to minimize the time that they experience symptoms (Ho et al 2000, Lieberman and Fenton 2000).

The delays that precede initial treatment for psychotic disorders are characterized by two phases:

- the prodromal period prior to the onset of obvious psychotic symptoms
- the period of undiagnosed and untreated psychosis

First-episode psychosis is most common in adolescents and young people. These individuals are particularly vulnerable to disruption of their developmental pathways. Consequences arising from delayed treatment for psychotic symptoms are listed in the text box.

Consequences of delayed treatment
- slower and less complete recovery
- poorer prognosis
- increased risk of depression and suicide
- interference with psychological and social development
- strain on relationships
- loss of family and social supports
- disruption of patient's parenting skills (for those with children)
- distress and increased psychological problems within the patient's family
- disruption of study and employment

- substance misuse
- violence/criminal activities
- unnecessary hospitalization
- loss of self-esteem and confidence
- increased cost of management

Early case detection in practice

The duration of untreated psychosis is an important indicator of efforts to improve the outcome in first-episode psychosis. Unlike other prognostic variables such as genetic vulnerability, gender and age of onset, the duration of untreated psychosis is potentially malleable and can be the focus of intervention strategies. Psychosis may be easier and less confusing to detect than schizophrenia (Driessen et al 1998, McGorry 1995a). Schizophrenia requires a period of frank psychotic features for diagnosis and may take time to emerge as a stable diagnosis. Instead, our primary treatment target is positive psychotic symptoms for which we prescribe antipsychotic medications.

The literature supports an association between the duration of untreated psychosis and initial response to treatment (Norman and Malla, 2001). The relationship between duration of untreated psychosis (DUP) and outcome at 1 year is equivocal – there are recent negative (e.g. Craig et al 2000, Ho and Andreasen 2000) and positive reports (e.g. Malla et al, in press). Johannessen (2001)

points out that patients with long DUP are more reluctant to enter studies and that this research bias has not been taken into account in studies which have failed to find a relationship between DUP and the course of first-episode psychosis. Assuming the link is robust, is the association causal? That is, does a delay in treatment actually contribute to a worse outcome, or is the link due to a common underlying factor such as a more severe form of illness, a more insidious onset, more negative symptoms, more paranoid ideation, less salience and awareness of change, or less willingness to seek and accept treatment?

Although it is not yet clearly proven that reducing the duration of untreated psychosis improves outcome, there is a strong prima facie case that delayed treatment is already a major public health problem. Patients and families suffer directly from the destructive effects of delay and the range of negative psychosocial outcomes that accumulate during the period of untreated psychosis.

Mental health services in partnership with local communities, primary care and individual clinicians, can embark on a range of strategies to reduce delays in accessing treatment. This is a novel concept for some clinicians and clinical services, and it is sometimes more common for services to attempt to limit their workload by restricting access by new patients. It is true that early detection strategies may lead to increased case loads, but the pattern of the work may also change:

- Intensive efforts to improve mental health literacy in the general community, recognition skills among general practitioners and access to specialist mental health services should reduce the duration of untreated psychosis for the average case. This should make the work of the service easier and result in a reduced need for inpatient care and involuntary treatment.
- There will be a reduction in the prevalence of hidden psychiatric morbidity in the community.

Strategies to reduce the duration of untreated psychosis are listed in the text box.

> **Strategies to reduce duration of untreated psychosis**
> - Improve recognition:
>   - educate primary care providers
>   - raise awareness of the early signs of psychosis
>   - educate the community – reduce the stigma associated with psychotic disorders, which can deter patients and their families from seeking help
> - Increase referrals:
>   - provide a responsive, user-friendly service

> - reduce the fear and stigma associated with psychiatric services
> - Provide easy access to psychiatric services:
>   - rapid response
>   - flexible approach
>   - assertive outreach

More resources will be required for services to become proactive, undertake the detection role and cope with the additional caseloads. Such a role should be expected of modern community-based mental health services and requires leadership from within psychiatry, but it needs to be developed in partnership with communities and primary care. It also needs to be considered in the budgets for health services.

Optimal management of the first episode and the critical period

Background

It is an attractive notion that optimal treatment of the early phase of psychosis might shorten the duration of illness and reduce the prevalence of the disorder, and also have a positive effect on the course and outcome. The 'critical period' follows recovery from a first episode of psychosis and extends for up to 5 years subsequently, and it is a phase of high vulnerability (Birchwood et al 1998). Optimal and sustained treatment during this critical period, when the vulnerability is at its peak, can provide a degree of 'damage control'. This strategy is supported by the fact that the level of disability attained within the first 2 years or so after entry to treatment strongly predicts the level of disability many years later.

Optimization and intensification of early treatment could be implemented and evaluated within mental health services even with the present level of knowledge. Given the alternative for patients and families, we really should ask, why not? Reducing the burden of disease during the period is worthwhile, even if it does not influence the ultimate level of disability. This is a highly appropriate treatment goal that is uncontroversial in other areas of health care, such as diabetes, rheumatoid arthritis and hypertension.

Optimal, intensive, phase-specific intervention

More intensive phase-specific treatment during the first episode of psychosis, and beyond into the critical period, involves less change in mind-set and service structures than prepsychotic intervention or early case detection. Whether it is possible to reduce the intensity of treatment over a longer time frame is an important but, as yet, unanswered

question. Recent studies suggest that treatment intensity should not be reduced within the first 5 years for the majority of patients.

Assessment and treatment of first-episode psychosis

Key elements of management in first-episode psychosis are briefly summarized below.

Access and engagement (see Chapter 3)

- Most people who develop psychotic disorders are young and have little or no experience of mental health services and carry the same fears and prejudices as the rest of the community about mental illness.
- Psychotic symptoms may further inhibit awareness and help-seeking.
- Engagement with services is more difficult if involuntary treatment is the initial experience of the young patient and family.
- Mobile assessment is a key advance in improving access to care.

Assessment (see Chapter 3)

- Assessment should be comprehensive, undertaken in a stepwise fashion so as not to undermine engagement.

- Initial assessment should focus on the diagnostic issues and levels of risk of harm to self or others.
- Substance misuse is frequent and it is important to identify the small proportion of cases where the psychosis represents an acute intoxication.
- Promotion of early detection will lead to the presentation of more subthreshold cases. Detection and diagnosis of psychosis, rather than the assignment of a precise DSM-IV or ICD-10 diagnosis, is an appropriate initial target.

Acute treatment (see Chapter 3)

- Where possible, home-based acute care is preferred.
- A full physical examination and medical assessment, including appropriate investigations, should be undertaken.
- An antipsychotic-free period of at least 48 hours is advisable, using benzodiazepines to alleviate agitation, anxiety and insomnia. If sustained psychosis is confirmed then antipsychotic medication can be commenced.
- The second-generation or novel antipsychotics are indicated as first-, second- and even third-line therapy because of their greater efficacy and better tolerability. The starting dose should be very low, with slow upward titration if needed.

- Emergency situations requiring urgent sedation can be managed with intravenous/intramuscular benzodiazepines such as midazolam or lorazepam. In some cases this will prove ineffective and a short-acting sedating antipsychotic is the next best option.
- Longer-acting depot preparations such as zuclopenthixol acetate might be thought worthwhile because repeated injections can be avoided. However, delayed action and almost inevitable distressing side effects outweigh the benefits.
- Intensive psychosocial support is essential for the patient and family.
- Identification and treatment of major affective syndromes, especially mania, is a key issue. A manic syndrome should be treated rapidly with a mood stabilizer to promote full recovery. Depression, unless clearly dominating the clinical picture, commonly resolves in parallel with the positive psychotic symptoms. If it persists or worsens during the postpsychotic period, it should be actively treated with a combination of antidepressants and psychological intervention.

The recovery phase (see Chapter 4)

- Up to 85–90% of first-episode patients will achieve a remission or partial remission of their positive psychotic symptoms within 12 months of initiation of treatment.

- A range of psychosocial strategies can augment the recovery process, including psychological intervention, family interventions and group-based recovery programmes.
- An integrated shared care model, involving the general practitioner and other agencies, is beneficial.
- The early course of schizophrenia and affective psychosis is turbulent and relapse prone with up to 80% of patients relapsing within 5 years. Drug therapy should be continued for most patients for at least 12 months after recovery from a first psychotic episode.

- Relapse prevention is not the sole consideration in treatment. Adaptation to illness is a challenging and often overwhelming task for these young people and they usually need to be given time and special help to come to an acceptance of the need for maintenance treatment.
- A concerted effort should be made to maintain the engagement of patients with clinical care and to have a written relapse plan so that action can be taken if symptoms re-emerge. A good therapeutic and personal relationship with the patient and family is the key to success and should be nurtured.

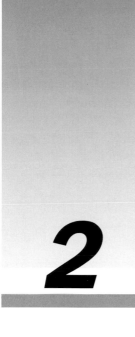

Key service elements – (a) early recognition and assistance

2

Triggers for considering psychosis or prepsychosis

The onset of psychotic disorders occurs most commonly in late adolescence or early adulthood. The possibility of a psychotic disorder should be considered when an adolescent or young person experiences a persistent and unexplained change in behaviour or functioning, particularly when other risk factors for a psychotic disorder are present. A family history of psychotic illness is one of the most important risk factors.

Signs and symptoms

Maintain a high index of suspicion

Early diagnosis of psychotic disorders and early intervention will be assisted by maintaining a high index of suspicion among the age groups most at risk. Signs and symptoms that may be associated with a psychotic illness include:

- a persistent change in psychosocial functioning, such as deterioration in work or study, withdrawal, loss of interest in socializing, and loss of energy or motivation

- behavioural changes such as sleep disturbances or altered appetite
- emotional change and other subjective experiences such as depression, anxiety, tension, irritability, anger, mood swings, a perception that things have changed, or beliefs that thoughts have speeded up or slowed down
- cognitive changes such as difficulties with memory or concentration, suspiciousness, and the emergence of unusual beliefs

These signs are not necessarily specific for a developing psychosis as they can also be caused by other disorders or be temporary reactions to stressful events. However, an unexplained reduction in adaptive functioning and loss of peer relationships in a young person is a key indicator for further assessment.

Positive psychotic symptoms

New-onset psychotic disorders are often first recognized when clear positive symptoms of psychosis emerge. Positive symptoms include thought disorder, delusions and hallucinations. Such symptoms often continue until the patient receives appropriate treatment, but in some cases they resolve spontaneously.

Risk factors

The presence of risk factors for psychotic illness should be assessed if a change in behaviour or functioning has been noticed. Risk factors can be divided into three main groups, as outlined in the text box.

Risk factors for psychotic illness
- age: adolescence and young adulthood
- trait risk factors:
  - family history of psychotic disorder
  - vulnerable personality (e.g. schizoid or schizotypal)
  - poor premorbid functioning
  - delayed milestones in childhood
  - history of head injury
  - low intelligence
  - history of obstetric or perinatal complications
  - winter birth
- state risk factors:
  - life events
  - perceived psychosocial stress
  - substance misuse
  - subjective and functional change

At-risk mental state

If an individual is experiencing signs and symptoms that might represent the early stages of a psychotic disorder, it can be useful to conceptualize the person as having an 'at-risk' mental state. In such individuals it is important to check for other features that may make the possibility of psychosis more likely, including the presence of the risk factors listed in the text box. Monitoring people identified as being at risk for transition to a fully fledged psychotic syndrome has been termed the 'close-in' strategy. For example, should a young person present with recent onset of depressed mood, poor motivation and deteriorating school performance, one would be more suspicious that a psychotic disorder was developing if the condition had been present for several weeks for no apparent reason and there was also a family history of schizophrenia.

Pathways to care

The pathway to appropriate care following the onset of a psychotic illness can be long, indirect and inefficient (Lincoln and McGorry 1999). For example, a study in the UK examined the pathways into the hospital system for people experiencing a first psychotic episode, from the point of view of the families (Johnstone et al 1986). It found that:

- Appropriate services were not available to relatives when required.

- Multiple contacts were made before admission.
- Relatives usually made appropriate contacts initially, but when these proved unsuccessful they were forced to turn to more unusual contacts.
- Police contact was distressing for relatives but they were grateful when it led to hospital admission.

Another study, in Australia, reviewed 62 people who had experienced a first episode of psychosis (Lincoln and McGorry 1995, Lincoln et al 1998). It found that:

- The mean number of helping contacts with a variety of professionals and nonprofessionals prior to referral to a specialist centre was 4.9 (range 1–17).
- 55% of people had four to six contacts.
- 16% had more than six helper contacts.
- 36% of initial help-seeking contacts were with a general practitioner (primary care physician) and 50% had seen a general practitioner at some stage prior to referral to the specialist centre.
- 50% were probably psychotic by the time they first sought help and another 37% were manic or depressed.

The pathway to care commonly involves a progression from non-psychiatric medical services (or even non-medical services) to psychiatric services, with general practitioners having a potentially important role in the early recognition and referral of individuals with early psychosis. The pathways to care are variable, depending on the nature of the health care system and its financial and structural characteristics. There is a significant prevalence of 'never-treated' psychosis, particularly in developing countries.

Factors associated with treatment delay

Difficulties in recognition

Although general practitioners are expected to identify conditions that occur at a low incidence in their patients, the detection of psychosis can present particular problems. The brevity of consultations, combined with a lack of experience and training in psychiatric interviewing, can mean that important features of mental state go unrecognized. For example, a failure to interview family members or to give enough weight to the information gleaned from them can mean that changes in behaviour or functioning are misinterpreted or regarded as unimportant.

The first signs of psychotic illness in young people can be misinterpreted by their families and friends as normal adolescent behaviour and may be tolerated for long periods before help is sought. Young people may, therefore, be particularly at risk of experiencing delays in accessing treatment. Families and friends may

also believe that the young person is going through a phase that will pass, or they may attribute the changed behaviour to character weakness or stress. The frequently insidious onset of psychotic disorders is another factor in delayed recognition by those around a young person. Promotion of mental health literacy, in which the general public becomes better informed about mental illness, could potentially improve the recognition of early psychotic symptoms and access to care.

Symptomatology can affect the likelihood and extent of treatment delay. Certain behavioural patterns such as mood disturbance and self-destructive acts appear to be more likely to trigger responses from the public and professionals. Patients with affective psychosis are subject to less delay than those with schizophrenia, perhaps because affective psychoses tend to have more florid symptoms.

Interpretation of changes in behaviour may be complicated by the overlapping of two separate processes (Eaton 1999). The first is intensification of pre-existing symptoms that may have been present for a long time or never have been absent (e.g. personality traits). The second is the emergence of new symptoms that did not exist before – that is, the acquisition of symptoms. As more symptoms emerge, they may form clusters that increasingly approach the threshold for fulfilling diagnostic criteria for a specific illness. It may take some time for subtle changes in behaviour or function to develop to sufficient severity so that they fulfil the definition of a 'disorder', even though the individual, family and others may have been aware that a problem existed.

Reluctance to seek help

Patients and their families can be reluctant to seek help for a variety of reasons, for example:

- poor knowledge of the features of mental disorders and their treatability
- denial that a problem exists
- belief that the problem can be solved without help
- magico-religious explanatory models of mental illness
- the stigma and shame associated with mental illness
- lack of confidence in health professionals and the treatments they provide
- lack of knowledge of resources
- trivializing or minimizing the severity of problems
- a desire to confine the problem within existing networks.

Factors such as gender, age, the perceived severity of symptoms and views of health professionals can all influence help-seeking behaviour. Adolescents can overestimate or underestimate the degree to which mental health professionals can help and may lack

confidence in their competence, preferring non-professional sources of help until these prove inadequate. They may expect doctors to know what their problem is, despite failing to explain it.

The negative stereotypes of mental illness, and the fear and stigma associated with mental health services, can inhibit help-seeking and lead to families denying symptoms or trying to manage abnormal behaviour for as long as possible. Seeking help is often seen as a last resort rather than a rational choice. Public acceptance of psychosis as a treatable condition would reduce the stigma associated with it.

General practitioners and other primary care professionals may also be inhibited from seeking specialist help because of factors such as:

- lack of knowledge about resources and how to access them
- disillusionment with mental health services
- a belief that patients and families may be offended by a suggestion of psychiatric help.

Inaccessible or non-responsive services

Services for the assessment and treatment of psychotic illnesses are frequently located in a psychiatric facility. Young people experiencing distressing changes in behaviour may be alarmed by the idea that these services could be relevant to them, or may be reluctant to incur the stigma associated with attending such a facility.

Some outpatient mental health services have long waiting lists. Existing services may be more comfortable managing known patients than new referrals, who may require more intensive assessment and follow up. The services may not be sufficiently focused on dealing with the early recognition of psychosis and its precursors, and may fail to follow up new referrals to ensure engagement in treatment. Additionally, a focus on patients with an established mental illness may mean that the early stages of potentially serious

Table 2.1
'Smooth' and 'rocky' pathways to recovery from psychosis

Smooth	Rocky
Early detection	*Late detection*
Treatment started rapidly	*Treatment started late*
Short duration of untreated psychosis	*Long duration of untreated psychosis*
Continual treatment	*Interrupted treatment*
Optimal treatment: medication, individual counselling, family support, psychosocial treatment, information	*Fragmented, inaccessible or incomplete care*
Supportive social network	*Little support from immediate environment*
Stable living environment	*Much stress and tension*
Structure and calm	*Conflictual personal relationships*
Meaningful occupations: study, work, hobby	*Idle times filled by worrying*
Someone to share experiences and feelings with	*Isolation and loneliness*
Good physical health	*Neglect of physical health and abuse of drugs*
Rapid disappearance of symptoms	*Persistent symptoms of psychosis and long-lasting disability, persistent depressive symptoms*
Lasting absence of symptoms	*Relapse of psychosis and recurrence of positive symptoms*
Realistic expectations and hope for the future	*Inadequate understanding of the illness, hopelessness*

Adapted with permission of EPO Publishing, from De Hert M, Magiels G, Thys E (2000) The Secret of the Brain Chip. *Antwerp, EPO Publishing*

mental illness is excluded – that is, patients' symptoms may have to become more severe and be associated with increased risks of sustained disability before they are given access to the service.

Groups at high risk for delayed treatment

Young homeless people are at particular risk for delayed treatment because they are often out of touch with relevant agencies or services may be hostile towards them. Those involved in substance misuse or who have personality disorders or intellectual disability may find that social or legal factors are a barrier to seeking care.

Table 2.1 illustrates the contrasts between 'smooth' and 'rocky' pathways to care.

Service developments – examples at EPPIC

Services can be designed to reduce delays in access to treatment and reduce secondary morbidity, while maximizing the number of high-risk people targeted and minimizing the number of false positives. Three strategies for early detection of young people at risk of developing psychoses currently operating at the Early Psychosis Prevention and Intervention Centre (EPPIC) in Melbourne, Australia, are outlined below.

Youth Access Team

The Youth Access Team (YAT; formerly the Early Psychosis Assessment Team, see Yung et al, 1999) is a multidisciplinary mobile assessment, crisis intervention and community treatment team which provides the first point of contact with EPPIC. It operates 24 hours per day, 7 days per week, to provide assessment for young people aged 15–29 years presenting with a first episode of psychosis and, if required, intensive home-based treatment. YAT uses networking and carefully targeted community education activities to raise community awareness of psychosis in young people and to promote recognition and early referral. Possible cases are always assessed in person, and referers are encouraged to re-refer if signs indicative of an early psychosis develop at a later point.

The team strives to minimize the stress involved in what is likely to be the first contact with psychiatric services by:

- providing information and support at each stage of the assessment phase

- being available to conduct assessments in the least threatening environment, for example in the home, school or local doctor's surgery
- responding flexibly to each situation

A major focus for the team is promoting the patient's engagement with treatment. For example, in cases in which a young person is likely to take several weeks to recognize the need for treatment and to develop sufficient motivation to attend regular appointments, home-based treatment and support can be provided. YAT also attempts to minimize the potential trauma involved in inpatient admissions and facilitates early discharge planning from inpatient care.

In the first 2 years of operation the team received 956 referrals for assessment of possible psychosis, of which 587 were clinically assessed and 398 were accepted into EPPIC, representing 80% of EPPIC's total intake for that period. About 40% of EPAT assessments took place at the young person's own home, and 21% at an agency that was not part of psychiatric services. In the first 6 months, 50% of referrals came from a non-psychiatric source, with 10% from family and friends. In the second 6 months, the figures increased to 69 and 25%, respectively, indicating that the community education programme was having an impact. About 5% of referrals came from general practitioners initially, increasing to nearly 10% with more intensive education. In the first 12 months of the service, the mean time between receiving a call for an urgent assessment and arriving for the assessment was 68 minutes; the mean response for non-urgent referrals was 3.1 days. Only 9% of all involuntary admissions required police transport.

Over the period July 2000 to June 2001, YAT received 3108 referrals for assessment of psychosis and common disorders, crisis intervention, and community treatment, reflecting an expanding role.

The Compass Project

Mental health literacy is defined as "the ability to recognise specific disorders; knowing how to seek mental health information; knowledge of risk factors and causes, of self-treatments, of professional help available; and attitudes that promote recognition and appropriate help seeking" (Jorm et al 1997, p. 182).

The Compass Project is a local community awareness campaign to promote early help-seeking for mental health problems. It is being implemented in metropolitan and rural settings (western Melbourne and the nearby Barwon region) and targets the 12- to 25-year age group. Compass builds on the experience of an early pilot project (Krstev et al 2001a) and aims to encourage early help-seeking through enhanced mental health literacy. It addresses:

- the public's knowledge of psychiatric disorders, particularly early signs of illness
- myths about mental illness and its treatment
- provision of information about the early symptoms of psychosis and mood disorder
- introduction of mental health service providers to the public, and methods for contacting them

Media communication strategies include advertisements for radio, newspaper and cinema; the youth press; a range of printed material; and a website (www.getontop.org/home.htm). Different strategies are used for young people and their families.

The development and implementation process has been guided by recommendations for public communication campaigns made by McGuire (1984) and Green and Kreuter (1999). These include:

- exploration of environmental and behavioural factors that influence early help-seeking
- clarification of predisposing, enabling and reinforcing factors that underpin help-seeking behaviour
- development of campaign material based on these findings and research in the area of effective communication strategies
- evaluation focusing on mental health literacy and help-seeking outcomes such as duration of untreated illness and treated incidence

Enquiries: compass@getontop.org

General practitioner–consultant liaison

General practitioners are often the first point of contact for young people seeking assistance for mental health problems and they play a critical role in ensuring that the delays in intervention are kept to a minimum (Hodges et al 1999). Early intervention programmes need to develop strong links with local general practitioners and their representative organizations. Strategies include:

- raising awareness and promoting interest in psychosis
- providing information about early intervention in psychosis
- education and training targeted at improving skills in psychiatric assessment, illness detection and treatment principles
- advice and support through outreach/liaison, psychiatric mentoring or clinical supervision (Carr and Donovan 1992, Falloon 1992, Falloon et al 1996)
- streamlining referral pathways between general practitioners and specialist services.

Divisions of General Practice
There is collaboration between EPPIC and three regional groupings of general practitioners known as Divisions of General Practice. Current activities include:

- a monthly newsletter providing practice updates on major mental disorders affecting young people
- continuing medical education workshops held monthly
- biannual intensive short courses on psychiatric interviewing and treatment skills
- an 'Associate Program' which involves outreach consultation to general practitioners, bimonthly group supervision and shared-care arrangements with the psychiatric service

These activities are supported by a range of resources in early psychosis including:

- two videos: *A Stitch in Time* (Ioannides and Hexter 1994a, 1994b, 1994c) and *Early Diagnosis of Psychosis* (Educational Resources Production Unit of the Royal Australian College of General Practitioners 1996), and a booklet (EPPIC 1994) for general practitioners
- a handbook, *Early Diagnosis and Management of Psychosis* (2001) and fact sheets (www.eppic.org.au)

Educational materials on early psychosis should reflect local circumstances (e.g. see the booklet and video for physicians developed through the Early Psychosis Initiative operating in British Columbia, Canada, described in Chapter 6).

Prodromal phase

What is the prodrome?

A period of behavioural or functional change prior to the onset of obvious psychotic symptoms is referred to as the prepsychotic prodrome. In most cases, the prodrome is defined retrospectively once a diagnosis of psychotic disorder has been made. The prodrome may be considered in two ways:

• the earliest form of a psychotic disorder
• a syndrome conferring increased vulnerability to psychosis – that is, an 'at-risk mental state' or 'precursor state' (Eaton et al 1995)

If the prodrome is indeed an early form of psychotic disorder then, in the absence of intervention, psychosis will inevitably follow. Alternatively, if the prodrome is a risk factor for psychosis, then only a proportion of individuals experiencing a prodrome will progress to a psychotic episode. It has been difficult to prospectively identify people experiencing a prodromal syndrome,

particularly because the features are variable and non-specific. However, information about the prodrome is starting to accumulate, and increased understanding of the syndrome has facilitated formation of a prospective framework to explain the development of psychosis and the potential of prevention (Yung and McGorry 1996).

Prodromal features most commonly described in first-episode psychosis are summarized in the text box.

Features of the prepsychotic prodrome (in descending order of frequency)
• reduced concentration, attention
• reduced drive and motivation, anergia
• depressed mood
• sleep disturbance
• anxiety
• social withdrawal
• suspiciousness
• deterioration in role functioning
• irritability

Symptoms of the prodrome for schizophrenia are prevalent in adolescents generally (Table 2.2), adding to the difficulties of prospective diagnosis. The prevalence of these symptoms suggests they are unlikely to be specific to the development of schizophrenia or other psychotic disorders.

Table 2.2
Prevalence of DSM-III-R schizophrenia prodrome symptoms in Australian 16-year-olds (rated as occurring occasionally or often)

Symptom	Presence (%)
Magical ideation	*51.0 (often, 9.3)*
Unusual perceptual experiences	*45.6 (often, 5.3)*
Social isolation/withdrawal	*18.4*
Markedly impaired role function	*41.1*
Blunted, flat or inappropriate affect	*21.7*
Digressive or over-elaborate speech	*21.7*
Marked lack of initiative or energy	*39.7*
Markedly peculiar behaviour	*25.2*
Marked impairment in personal hygiene	*8.1*

*Adapted with permission, from McGorry PD, McFarlane C, Patton GC et al (1995) The prevalence of prodromal features of schizophrenia in adolescence: a preliminary survey. Acta Psychiatr Scand **92**:241–249.*

Prodromal features may be considered precursors to, or an at-risk mental state for, a range of disorders including psychoses. In one study (Jackson et al 1995), individuals with a diagnosis of schizophrenia had a significantly higher proportion of prodromal symptoms than people in the other diagnostic groups, although these symptoms were not exclusive to schizophrenia. In general, individual prodromal symptoms predicted up to around 50% of cases of schizophrenia and up to 20% of cases of schizophreniform disorder. Although prodromal symptoms are specified in DSM-III-R for schizophrenia, they are not specified for other psychotic diagnoses and were dropped from DSM-IV.

A two-stage screening process may be helpful in identifying and interpreting prodromal features (McGorry 2000; McGorry et al 2001b). Individuals at high risk of psychosis can be identified by features that include attenuated psychotic symptoms, brief limited intermittent psychotic symptoms, or trait and state factors, which include a strong family history of psychotic disorder, the presence of schizotypal personality disorder or significant decrease in mental functioning. Individuals with one or more of these features have a 30–40% of developing a psychotic illness, compared with a risk of less than 1% in the general population of adolescents and young adults. A second stage of screening involves close observation and follow up of individuals identified as being at increased risk.

The duration of untreated psychosis is

long, with patients typically experiencing symptoms for 1 or 2 years before accessing treatment (Johannessen et al 1999). Patients with schizophrenia also commonly have a long period of prepsychotic prodromal symptoms before the onset of psychosis, ranging from 1 to 5 years (Larsen et al 2000a).

What happens in the prodromal phase?

Effects of the prodrome include:

- profound changes in subjective experience and behaviour including isolation from families and friends, damage to social and working relationships and prospects, deviant behaviour causing crises and losses, and increased risk of self-harm, aggression and substance misuse
- changes in sense of self and maturation of personality, leading to aberrant development which may be difficult to reverse

A hybrid/interactive model has been proposed (Yung and McGorry 1996) in which a person moves in and out of periods of non-specific symptoms and periods of attenuated psychotic symptoms. Both types of symptoms may result in behavioural changes.

Intervention in the prodrome

The variety of non-specific symptoms that may be present during the prodrome and their high prevalence in the general population of adolescents and young adults means that there is a substantial risk of 'false positives' and unnecessary intervention in individuals who would not have progressed to a psychotic illness. Until further information is gathered about the prodromal state itself, the relative risks of progression to psychosis, and the nature of this transition, the use of preventive strategies must remain limited. Nevertheless, there are a number of approaches that can be recommended despite the current limitations in our understanding. They include:

- *Early recognition and access to care:* young people experiencing pervasive emotional and behavioural changes, particularly when these are persistent, need easy access to expert assessment. Efforts should be directed at parents, health professionals (particularly general practitioners) and teachers to raise their awareness of these changes in young people, with a view to promoting earlier recognition and assessment.
- *Follow up of at-risk groups:* young people considered at high risk can be offered follow up and appropriate intervention. High risk may be indicated by features such as more severe symptoms, a rapid rate

of change of symptoms, or the presence of other risk factors such as substance misuse or family history. Intervention can address issues such as the distress associated with subthreshold psychotic symptoms, or specific risk factors such as substance misuse. Close follow up should minimize the delay in diagnosis and treatment of those who do develop florid psychosis.

Future research should facilitate the identification of individuals who would benefit from 'preventive' treatment with antipsychotics and other forms of medication before the emergence of florid psychosis. At present, this cannot be widely recommended because of the rate of false-positive cases. However, psychosocial intervention is justified to reduce the level of symptoms and disability in this group (Yung et al 1996).

Personal Assessment and Crisis Evaluation

The Personal Assessment and Crisis Evaluation (PACE) clinic was established at EPPIC to identify and treat individuals who are thought to be at imminent risk of developing a psychotic disorder (McGorry et al 2001a, Yung et al 1995, 1996; www.pace-clinic.org). Offices are located at a generalist adolescent health centre and a suburban

shopping complex in order to avoid premature 'labelling' and stigmatization. Intake criteria were guided by a pilot phase of research and clinical experience (Phillips et al 2000). Young people were identified as being at possible risk of a psychotic illness on the basis of one or more of the following:

- family history of psychotic illness or a DSM-IV schizotypal personality disorder and a recent change in mental state *or*
- subthreshold psychotic symptoms (such as unusual perceptual experiences) occurring several times a week over a period of at least 1 week *or*
- brief, limited or intermittent psychotic symptoms (BLIPS) lasting less than a week and which spontaneously remit

The rate of transition to psychosis in a pilot study was 41% at 12 months and more than 50% at 24 months. In a larger sample using the same criteria, transition to psychosis occurred in 35% of cases (Yung et al in press).

Assessment, monitoring, support and referral are provided. Psychological interventions (McGorry et al 1998) and medical treatments are offered with the aim of ameliorating symptoms, enhancing coping strategies, and ultimately – it is hoped – delaying or preventing the onset of psychosis. The clinic undertakes research on the prediction of psychosis (Yung et al 1998a, 1998b) and the outcomes of intervention (McGorry et al in press).

Between March 1995 and January 1999, PACE received 690 referrals, of whom 196 met inclusion criteria. Patients accepted by PACE have higher mean scores on general psychopathology and negative symptom measures and experience greater disability than patients recovering from a first episode of psychosis (Yung et al 1996).

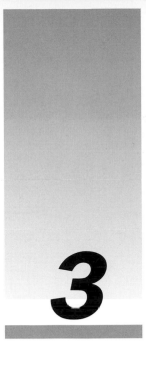

Key service elements – (b) initial assessment and treatment

3

This chapter provides a brief introduction to the initial assessment and treatment of individuals with a first episode of psychosis. A detailed description is beyond the scope of this book, but several excellent references are available if further information is required:

- Aitchison et al (1999)
- McGorry and Jackson (1999; Chapters 6–8)

Assessment procedures for first-episode psychosis

Engagement

Assessment procedures for patients experiencing their first episode of psychosis should incorporate strategies to promote engagement. For most patients, this will be their first experience of the mental health system. They will usually have little knowledge or understanding of mental illness in general, or their illness in particular, and they may be fearful of the illness and the prospect of treatment. Some techniques for promoting engagement are highlighted in the text box.

Engagement techniques

- Recognize that the patient may be nervous, wary or not want to see health professionals.
- Be aware that psychosis may distort patients' mode of interaction and their ability to process information (e.g. constant auditory hallucination may impair concentration).
- Listen carefully to patients and take their views seriously.
- Acknowledge and respect the patient's viewpoint.
- Identify common ground.
- Consider what is appropriate body language when interviewing a patient who may be paranoid, aroused or manic:
  - sit side-by-side (not too close) rather than face-on
  - avoid too much eye contact
  - allow personal space, for example walk around while talking
- Be helpful, active and flexible.
- Carefully explain the procedures involved in physical or other assessments.
- Gather information gradually, at the same time as fostering a close relationship.

- Introduce key players who will take part in the patient's ongoing management.
- Aim to provide continuity of care and good communication between professionals.

Engagement techniques may need to be tailored to the specific needs and expectations of young people, for example by using everyday language and common points of reference.

Psychiatric history

The following areas should be covered when taking a history from a patient presenting with a psychotic episode:

- Phenomenology – for example, what changes and new experiences has the patient noticed? What have others noticed? When did the patient and others think the symptoms had become serious enough to be considered 'abnormal'?
- Secondary symptoms – for example, what other symptoms or difficulties have arisen as a result of the psychotic changes?
- Course, duration and fluctuation – for example, when did symptoms first start? Are they getting better or worse? Do they change from day to day or week to week?

- Prodromal symptoms – for example, were any changes in experience, thoughts or behaviour noticed before it was clear that the patient was ill?
- Precipitants – for example, have there been recent stressors, life events, or initiation or change in drug use?
- Relieving factors and coping strategies – for example, what helps relieve the symptoms? What has the patient done to feel better?
- Any treatments already tried – did they help?
- Physical conditions potentially related to symptoms, including drug and alcohol use.
- Family history – is there any family history of psychotic or other mental illness? Does the family have any pre-existing ideas about treatment? What are the dynamics within the family? Are there psychological risks stemming from the family situation?
- Personal history – including full medical and social history in addition to any history of mental illness.
- Premorbid level of functioning.

Wherever possible, and with the patient's consent, relatives and friends should be interviewed by the clinician. Relatives and friends are often distressed, so the clinician should be empathic in the process of obtaining information and also attempt to deal with the needs of a family in crisis.

Important contextual factors and influences to be considered in the assessment process include:

- understanding the individual's specific needs, risks and issues in relation to a first episode of psychosis
- understanding the range of patients' reactions to psychosis, their personality structure, phase of development, defence style, coping skills and self-concept
- understanding the social and cultural milieu of the patient
- understanding patient and family attitudes to services and treatments
- understanding the impact of psychosis on the lives of patients and families
- appreciating the impact of premorbid intelligence, especially verbal abilities, on the patient's expression of psychosis

Risk assessment

Risks will vary with individuals but the following should be assessed as a starting point:

- suicide/self-harm
- severe self-neglect and death
- violence, aggression
- victimization by others
- non-adherence to treatment
- if an inpatient, leaving hospital prematurely

- substance misuse
- health risks (e.g. through unprotected sex)

- contributing or
- consecutive

to the psychosis.

Physical assessment

A full physical examination and medical assessment, including appropriate investigations, should be undertaken in patients who present with a first episode of psychosis. These are essential steps in working towards a diagnosis of the psychotic disorder, and also in ensuring the general health of the patient who may be at increased risk of accompanying physical diseases. Thus, physical disease may be:

- causal
- concomitant

Some physical illnesses that may produce psychotic symptoms or mimic psychotic disorders are listed in Table 3.1. Wherever possible, it is important to exclude these physical illnesses before initiating treatment for a functional psychosis (i.e. a psychotic illness that cannot be explained by physical causes). Investigations to be considered routinely in patients who appear to be experiencing a first episode of psychosis, and those to be considered in special circumstances, are summarized in Table 3.2.

Table 3.1
Some physical conditions associated with a higher risk of psychosis

---

Cushing's syndrome
Thyroid and parathyroid disorders
Cerebral sarcoidosis
Systemic lupus erythematosus
HIV–AIDS
Sex chromosome abnormalities
Demyelinating diseases such as multiple sclerosis and Schilder's disease
Encephalitic diseases such as cerebral syphilis and herpes simplex encephalitis
Wilson's disease
Huntington's disease
Friedreich's ataxia
Vitamin B12 deficiency
Subarachnoid haemorrhage
Cerebral tumours

Information obtained from Power and McGorry, 1999 (pages 155–183).

Table 3.2
Physical investigations in first-episode psychosis

Recommended as routine, before commencing antipsychotic medication
Urine tests:
    Drug screen
    General urine microscopy
Blood tests:
    Full blood evaluation
    Erythocyte sedimentation rate
    Renal function tests (urea, creatinine)
    Electrolytes
    Serum calcium and phosphate
    Liver function tests
    Thyroid function tests

Recommened as routine, as early as possible
Computed tomography brain scan or, ideally, magnetic resonance imaging scan
Electroencephalogram

Optional, depending on clinical circumstances
Urine tests:
    Pregnancy test
    Urinary porphyrins
Blood tests:
    Pregnancy test
    Fasting blood glucose
    Nutritional indices (B12, folate, iron studies)
    Autoantibody screens
    Hepatitis screens
    HIV and syphilis screens
    Copper studies
Imaging:
    Chest radiograph
    Electrocardiogram

Adapted with permission of Cambridge University Press, from Power and McGorry, 1999 (pages 155–183)

Diagnostic assessment

It is often difficult to determine a precise diagnosis early in the course of a first episode of psychosis. Psychotic syndromes can include a variety of symptoms, and may be accompanied by symptoms of comorbid illnesses. The pattern of symptoms can alter markedly over time. Fluid combinations of symptoms might be best understood as dimensions of psychopathology within broad categories of illness. Some specific forms of psychosis are listed in the text box.

Specific forms of psychosis:

- affective psychoses, including bipolar disorder (manic phase with psychotic features) and major depression with psychotic features
- schizophrenia
- schizoaffective disorder
- schizophreniform disorder
- brief reactive psychosis
- drug-induced psychosis
- medical or neurological illnesses mimicking primary psychiatric disorders

---

The diagnostic assessment made on initial contact with mental health services should be repeated after the patient has stabilized. Because of changes in symptoms and the refinement of diagnosis that often occurs in the early years of a psychotic illness, reassessment should also occur 1 and 2 years after the first episode. Relapses, comorbidities or persistent symptoms can be taken into account during the 'evolution' of a diagnosis.

Diagnostic instruments for first-episode psychosis

Although there are a wide variety of psychiatric assessment instruments, few have been developed specifically for first-episode psychosis. The Royal Park Multidiagnostic Instrument for Psychosis (RPMIP) was designed for the assessment of patients during an initial psychotic episode (McGorry et al 1990a, 1990b). It covers a large number of psychotic diagnoses and uses a multidiagnostic approach, including repeated interviews and multiple information sources. Häfner and colleagues (1992) developed the Interview for the Retrospective Assessment of the Onset of Schizophrenia (IRAOS) to allow assessment of symptoms, psychological impairments, demographic and social characteristics, and time course of the early episodes of psychosis. It uses a semistructured interview with the patient and a key informant, supplemented by examination of previous case notes.

Principles of initial treatment

"Detecting an illness early is of value only if effective treatment is readily available" (Falloon et al 1998, p. 33)

The aims of treatment of first psychotic episode are:

- remission of positive psychotic symptoms
- prevention, or early recognition and treatment, of comorbid symptoms including:
  - negative symptoms, particularly secondary negative symptoms
  - depression
  - mania/hypomania (common and poorly recognized in adolescents and young adults)
  - anxiety, panic attacks, post-traumatic stress disorder
  - substance misuse
- promotion of adjustment and psychosocial recovery in the face of disruptive, stigmatizing and often highly traumatic experiences during the key developmental phase of adolescence or early adulthood
- working with family and friends to provide support and encourage a good environment for the establishment and maintenance of recovery

Strategies for treatment of a first psychotic episode include:

- reducing delay in accessing treatment
- minimizing trauma, especially that associated with seclusion and restraint
- promoting engagement and the development of a therapeutic relationship
- commencing low-dose antipsychotic medication, using an atypical antipsychotic
- developing a common understanding of what has occurred (an 'explanatory model')
- developing a plan for crisis intervention
- supporting the family
- promoting functional recovery and good quality of life
- preventing maladaptive coping, for example substance misuse or deliberate self-harm

Associated or secondary conditions

People recovering from psychosis may present with a range of associated or comorbid syndromes such as:

- post-traumatic stress disorder
- panic disorder
- substance misuse
- obsessive–compulsive disorder
- insomnia
- depression
- social phobia

Sometimes it is difficult to disentangle pre-existing conditions from a condition that is secondary to psychosis (Jackson et al 2000, McGorry et al 1991).

The experience of a psychotic episode itself can also result in secondary morbidity for a number of reasons including:

- terrifying delusions or hallucinations leading to post-traumatic stress disorder
- fear and demoralization in the face of the psychotic disorder
- disruption of personality development
- loss of self-esteem and confidence
- the development of an unfavourable 'possible self'
- disruption of relationships with family and friends

Factors that may influence the emergence of these conditions include:

- the location of treatment
- the circumstances of admission to hospital
- traumatic events during treatment (e.g. distressing contact with other patients)
- the use of interventions such as seclusion or forced sedation
- relationships with staff
- side effects of medication

Techniques to reduce secondary morbidity include flexible arrangements for assessment of patients (which may allow contact with psychiatric institutions to be avoided), treatment at home when possible, and minimization of police involvement in admission. Medication strategies should minimize side effects, including extrapyramidal symptoms (which should now be considered as avoidable and unacceptable), hyperprolactinaemia, excessive weight gain, impaired glucose tolerance and diabetes.

Medication

The first experience of medication may strongly influence a patient's future attitudes to therapy of all types. People experiencing a first psychotic episode are often suspicious or frightened about the prospect of 'mind-altering' drugs. However, if medication provides relief from symptoms without severe adverse effects, patients are more likely to be reassured about its use and to collaborate in future therapy.

Several approaches can be helpful in persuading the patient (and the family) to accept drug treatment for the illness:

- Gently elicit fears about taking medication and provide appropriate information.
- Provide a temporary rationale for taking the medication:
  - as one element of a complete programme
  - to 'see if it helps' with symptoms such as stress, sleep disturbances, the impact of voices or feelings of persecution

A quantitative measure of symptom severity, such as the Brief Psychiatric Rating Scale-expanded (BPRS-E; Lukoff et al, 1986), is important so that the success of interventions can be assessed accurately.

Some prescribing principles are outlined in the text box and in Figures 3.1 and 3.2.

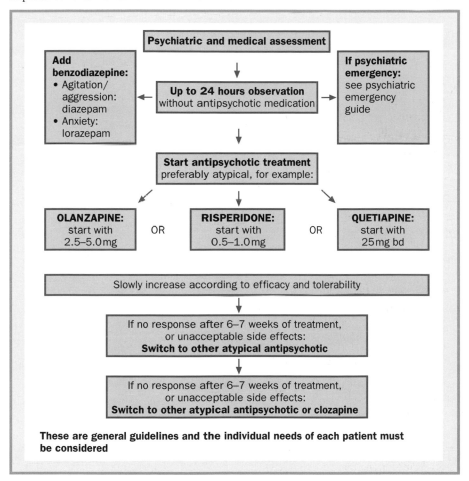

Figure 3.1
Non-affective first-episode psychosis – EPPIC pharmacotherapy guide.
Adapted with permission of Early Psychosis Prevention and Intervention Centre, Melbourne, from EPPIC (2002c).

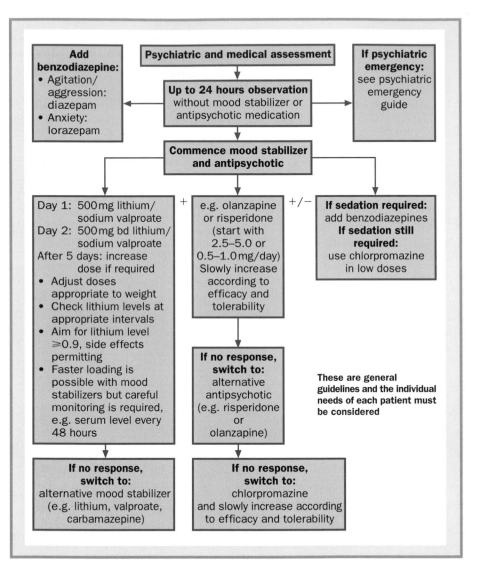

Figure 3.2
First-episode manic psychosis – EPPIC pharmacotherapy guide.
Adapted with permission of Early Psychosis Prevention and Intervention Centre, Melbourne, from EPPIC (2002c).

Prescribing principles in first-episode psychosis

- Maximize therapeutic benefit and minimize side effects.
- Use very low starting doses, particularly in patients not previously treated with antipsychotics.
- Adjust doses in small increments at appropriately spaced intervals, for example every 3 weeks.
- Review medication if symptoms worsen or the patient becomes suicidal.
- Have patience, as remission often takes several months.
- Consider short-term lithium treatment (3–6 months) for manic symptoms.
- Use benzodiazepines liberally to treat anxiety, agitation and insomnia in the acute phase.
- Consider antidepressants to treat depression.
- Use only one antipsychotic medication at a time.

Increasing the dose of an antipsychotic beyond a certain threshold does not necessarily confer any additional benefits (McEvoy et al 1991, Remington et al 1998). High doses increase the risk of side effects,

which may reduce adherence with the medication and therefore diminish the prospects of recovery. Prospective studies have confirmed that it can take several weeks to achieve a response to treatment and many months for remission to occur. For example, in a 5-year study of treatment response and outcome in first-episode schizophrenia, the mean interval between starting medication and achieving maximum improvement was 36 weeks, with a median of 11 weeks (Lieberman et al 1993). Less information is available on the time course of response for newer atypical antipsychotics.

Antipsychotic medication that maintains or improves cognitive function after a first psychotic episode, rather than impairing it, is likely to assist acquisition of insight, adherence to therapy, recovery and reintegration into society. Use of conventional antipsychotics, particularly at higher doses, can impair cognitive function but there is evidence that this is also impaired in patients treated with clozapine, olanzapine and risperidone (Harvey and Keefe 2001).

Long-term outcomes appear to be superior in patients treated with atypical rather than conventional antipsychotics. For example, one study showed that individuals with first-episode schizophrenia who had been treated with risperidone for more than 1 year had a significantly shorter length of first hospitalization, lower utilization of inpatient beds during the course of treatment and lower use of anticholinergic medication than a matched sample treated with only one conventional antipsychotic throughout the course of their illness (Malla et al 2001b).

Patients with early psychosis are at risk of over-treatment with antipsychotics if other symptomatic interventions are not considered. For example, lithium can be used to treat comorbid manic features (3–6 months' treatment), or aggression and overactivity (several weeks' treatment). This strategy can help reduce antipsychotic doses and may also prove to be neuroprotective (Manji et al 2000). Antidepressants can be used for postpsychotic depression and for mood-congruent psychotic depression.

Antipsychotic-free period

Although early assessment and care is an important objective in first-episode psychosis, an initial medication-free period is feasible in some patients who are not unduly distressed by their symptoms. A period free from medication may help clinicians to gain patients' trust, and promote better adherence to medication if it should become necessary. It also allows clinical investigations that may be influenced by medication, including electroencephalography (EEG) and magnetic resonance imaging (MRI), to be performed in the absence of such effects. A common consequence of late presentation is that patients may be too distressed or at too great a

risk for a medication-free period to be possible.

Prior to starting antipsychotics, benzodiazepines can be used (at moderate to high doses if needed) to treat anxiety for the first few days until a patient is more settled. Sedatives can be used for sleep disturbance. Intoxicated patients should be treated with caution because of possible drug interactions and the risk of respiratory depression. Organic conditions should also be treated carefully because of the possibility of masking neurological signs and the risk of paradoxic drug reactions.

Cognitive–behavioural therapy

Cognitive–behavioural therapy has been used increasingly to treat psychotic symptoms in patients with chronic schizophrenia and medication-resistant symptoms, but its use in acute or first-episode psychosis has not been extensively researched (Garety et al 2000). Drury et al (1996a, 1996b) conducted a small randomized controlled trial in acute inpatients, some of whom were experiencing first-episode psychosis. Patients were randomly assigned to either cognitive–behavioural therapy, consisting of individual sessions, group work and family sessions, or a control treatment provided by the same therapists. The results suggested that the cognitive–behavioural therapy hastened the relief of symptoms by 25–50%

(depending on the definition of recovery used) and halved the time spent in hospital. The study was not blinded, and it is not clear whether the intervention and control groups were comparable (Johnson 1996). Nevertheless, these results were consistent with studies of early medication that suggest that early intervention leads to better outcome. Drury has since elaborated on a cognitive–behavioural approach for the acute phase of early psychosis (Drury 2000).

The Study of Cognitive Reality Alignment Therapy in Early Schizophrenia (SOCRATES) was a multicentre, controlled psychological trial in people with schizophrenia who were experiencing a first or second psychotic episode and required admission to day care or inpatient care (Haddock et al 1998). The 316 participants were randomly allocated within 14 days of admission to one of three treatment conditions in addition to routine care: a standardized package of cognitive–behavioural therapy over 5 weeks, supportive counselling or no extra treatment. Results suggested that cognitive–behavioural therapy accelerated improvements in delusions and hallucinations, and that benefits were maintained beyond the acute phase (Lewis et al 2001a, 2001b).

Integrating care

Biological, social and psychological interventions must be integrated to provide maximum benefit to the patient. Treatment priorities will vary over the course of the illness, and a flexible approach is essential.

Medication is the basis of biological interventions, and the principles have been described above. Psychological approaches should aim to:

• explain the effects and side effects of medication and provide an acceptable rationale for its use
• provide reassurance and support
• develop a clear picture of the patient's experience of being psychotic and avoid traumatic procedures (e.g. forced sedation and seclusion)
• provide psychoeducation

Techniques to address the social issues related to the psychotic illness include:

• involvement with the family (and peers where appropriate) to provide support to them, educate them about the illness and its treatment, and facilitate their support of the patient
• assisting with practical problems, including finances, housing, and employment or educational commitments

Location of acute treatment

Home-based treatment

The resources and needs of the family, patient and care team must be carefully assessed when deciding whether a patient with a first episode of psychosis can be managed at home.

For the family, the following should be considered:

- the time available to provide care, taking into account work and other commitments
- the extent of a supportive network of family and friends
- relationships and interactions within the family
- the ability of the family to contain the individual and cope with risks, including suicidality and substance misuse

The family will need clear management plans, reassurance about the likely outcome, clear explanations about the management of the patient, and education regarding the illness.

For the individual, the following should be considered:

- the dangerousness of symptoms, rather than severity of illness
- the presence and extent of substance misuse
- potential danger within the home (e.g. access to weapons)

- the individual's role in the family
- attitudes to treatment

The care team needs to assess (Fitzgerald and Kulkarni 1998):

- the ability of the team to provide care as guests in the person's home
- whether they have sufficient experience and confidence to make independent decisions
- whether all members can function in specialty roles and also as generic clinicians
- whether staffing levels permit up to three visits per day
- whether the team is large enough to provide flexibility, with careful rostering
- whether continuous care can be maintained once the therapeutic alliance between clinician, patient and family has developed
- the ability to perform physical investigations
- issues of patient confidentiality, given the role of the family as care givers

The development of a treatment plan can be useful in giving carers and patients an idea of what to expect. This can take the form of a written timetable, setting out the interventions and processes that will occur at each stage. Confidence, optimism and pragmatism are the keys to successful psychoeducation in this setting.

Home treatment at EPPIC

At EPPIC, home-based treatment is undertaken by YAT (see Chapter 2) and follows similar principles to those of the Home-Oriented Management of Early Psychosis programme described by Fitzgerald and Kulkarni (1998).

Hospital-based treatment

If hospitalization is required, the following measures may be of benefit:

- separation of first-episode patients from older, chronically ill patients
- development of low-stigma settings
- clear explanation about admission and other procedures
- education about the roles of various professionals
- flexible visiting times
- attention to personal comfort and individual needs and requests
- privacy within the unit
- information about expected length of stay
- a facility for relatives to stay in the same unit overnight, particularly for younger patients

The EPPIC Inpatient Unit

The EPPIC Inpatient Unit provides acute treatment for patients who cannot be managed in the community because of a risk of self-harm or violence, refusal or inability to comply with assessment or treatment, or a lack of adequate support in the community.

The focus of the 16-bed facility is on symptom reduction and containment, emphasizing brief admission in order to prepare the person for community treatment either by YAT (see Chapter 2) or the outpatient case management service (see Chapter 4). This role is facilitated by staff members working across the different components of the programme and the immediate assignment of the case manager at entry to the programme. Median length of stay in the unit, adjusted for leave days, is currently 9 days for first admissions (mean 13.2 days) and 6 days for subsequent admissions.

Low doses of antipsychotics are standard practice during the acute phase. Disturbed behaviour is managed by targeted intensive nursing interventions, use of benzodiazepines and lithium as 'antipsychotic-sparing' agents, and minimizing the use of potentially traumatic interventions such as seclusion and restraint.

At least one-third of EPPIC patients are managed without requiring inpatient admission during the first 3 months of treatment (Power et al 1998), even though those treated in the community appear to be as unwell at initial presentation as those who are hospitalized. The level of social support available to supervise people in the community is a factor influencing admission. In general, both inpatients and those managed in the community are treated with low doses of antipsychotics, with a mean dose of 4.1 mg/day haloperidol equivalents (s.d. = 2.5, range 0.5–15.0 mg/day) and favourable reductions in symptoms. By the end of 3 months, 63% of a representative subsample were in remission.

Information gathered from a more recent EPPIC cohort suggested that almost half of the young people avoided admission during the first 3 months of treatment; approximately 36% avoided admission at any time over their 18-month period of care (Edwards et al, in press a).

Key service elements – (c) promoting recovery

4

Early intervention does not simply involve 'bringing forward' best practice to this early phase; it requires special care in recognition of the biological, psychological and familial challenges and changes that are active in this period. (Spencer et al 2001, p. 139)

Management of the recovery process after a first episode of psychosis aims to help patients reconstruct and reorient their lives, and assist them in understanding psychosis and develop resources for the future. Birchwood and Macmillan (1993) have proposed the concept of a 'critical period' extending for 2–5 years after a first psychotic episode, in which personal, social and biological factors influence the future balance between illness and well-being (see also Birchwood 1999, 2000). Most disability associated with psychotic illness develops in the first few years but then tends to plateau, and the level of functioning 2 years after a diagnosis predicts the level of functioning at 15 years. There are three propositions essential to the concept of the 'critical period':

- The course of psychosis is most 'stormy' at the onset and early in its course, plateauing thereafter.

- The biological, psychosocial and cognitive changes that are influential in the course of psychosis actively develop during this period.
- Interventions must focus on symptoms but should also focus on the psychosocial and psychological domains.

Concept of recovery

Since the time of Kraepelin (1896), concepts of schizophrenia have included an assumption that the illness is chronic and the prospects of recovery are slim. In fact, schizophrenia and other psychotic disorders are characterized by a wide range of outcomes, although outcomes are difficult to predict at the point of initial diagnosis and treatment. Individuals will probably be changed by the experience of psychosis, but this does not mean they cannot recover (McGorry 1992). The conventional rehabilitation model applies to patients in a relatively stable state who have skill deficits that need to be repaired or replaced in order for them to function normally. However, a more dynamic concept and therapeutic approach is required when considering early psychosis (Edwards et al 1994). Features of the recovery process are summarized in the text box.

Features of the recovery process

- Psychotic symptoms can subside relatively rapidly with medication, but in some cases this may take several months. The concept of 'relapse' is categorical (i.e. relapse either occurs or does not occur) and is a poor way of describing the fluctuations in symptoms that can occur during recovery.
- Recovery is a convalescent period of recuperation and readjustment.
- Recovery is an active process for patients and their families.
- As part of recovery, patients should develop an understanding of what has happened to them, integrate the experience and restore self-esteem.
- There may be a plateau in recovery when little appears to be happening, described as 'wood-shedding', 'moratoria', 'regrouping' or 'holding patterns' (Strauss et al 1985). This may reflect a period when the person is struggling with subtle psychotic symptoms or has been depressed or 'shut down'.
- For some people, a rapid return to their normal environment and responsibilities is helpful and may

minimize stigma and inappropriate illness behaviour. For others, there is a risk of precipitating a second episode of psychosis if reintegration is too rapid. Predicting the best approach is difficult. An insidious onset of illness and a long duration of untreated psychosis with slow remission may suggest that a gentle reintegration is preferable.

- For some people a paced approach is appropriate, with one stressor or step tackled at a time in working towards realistic and achievable goals.

Understanding the likely time to remission of symptoms may reduce the impatience felt by the patient, clinician and carers about the pace of recovery. Lieberman et al (1993) reported that the mean interval between initiating medication and achieving maximum improvement was 36 weeks, with a median of 11 weeks. About 80% of patients with first-episode psychosis will achieve full remission of positive symptoms within 6 months of starting treatment (Lieberman et al 1993, Szymanski et al 1996, Tohen et al 1992). It should be recognized that frequent relapses, worsening symptoms or exacerbating factors such as substance misuse will slow recovery

and add to the frustration of patients and their carers.

Assessment of recovery should take account of three separate elements: impairment (the characteristic symptoms of the illness), disability (the functional limitations experienced by the patient) and handicap (the disadvantage experienced by the patient in fulfilling normal roles such as student, worker, friend or family member). Where possible, levels of disability and handicap should be estimated and monitored. In general, medication has its greatest direct effect at the level of impairment, while psychosocial factors are targeted at the level of disability and handicap (McGorry, 1992).

It is important to establish a reliable picture of the patient's level of functioning prior to the onset of acute illness, so that premorbid limitations are not misinterpreted as failure to recover. For example, social underachievement often precedes the onset of psychotic symptoms in patients who later develop schizophrenia (Jones et al 1993). Definition of premorbid functioning is complicated by the possibility that the patient may have experienced a prolonged prodromal phase, making it difficult to define the true capacity for recovery. Because the first onset of psychotic illness is often in adolescence or early adulthood, the expectations for recovery should also take account of the anticipated developmental trajectory of patients: that is, the level of functioning they would have achieved if their development had not been interrupted by prodromal symptoms and the illness itself.

Phases of illness

An episode of psychosis can be divided into stages:

- prodrome
- acute phase, including clear emergence of psychotic symptoms
- early recovery
- late recovery

Patients have different therapeutic needs at different stages. Although the stages may overlap to some extent, separating recovery from the acute phase can facilitate the development and targeting of specialist services. Patients with acute psychosis generally require medication and a low-stimulation, highly supportive environment, which may be the family home. Recovering patients benefit from a more active approach including cognitive, psychotherapeutic and skill-based therapies.

Early recovery

Management of the early stage of recovery should focus on monitoring progress and creating the opportunity for patients to understand their experience of illness. It is helpful to adopt a gradual approach to

understanding the patient's life. Patients often create an idealized view of their premorbid selves, and they may need some time to adjust their perceptions to a more realistic view of their lives before the illness.

Differentiation of self from psychosis is critical in a young person seeking to establish identity. This differentiation can be promoted through careful use of language, for example, "You have experienced a psychotic episode" rather than "You are psychotic". In addition, it is helpful to develop experiences and areas of functioning (e.g. recreational or occupational) that are distinct from the psychosis so that patients rediscover things that they *can* do. Considerable time and effort may be required to discover these preserved areas of function and then to help patients to overcome financial, social or other barriers to resuming their activities (Edwards et al 1999).

Reintegration of a sense of self during early recovery includes re-establishment of family, school or work relationships. This will need continued provision of individual and family support, for example coping strategies and psychoeducation in a collaborative relationship between the clinicians, patient and family.

Late recovery

'Late recovery' refers to a period usually commencing about a year after the first onset of psychosis. Most first-episode patients will have recovered from their acute symptoms at this point. One prospective study of 118 first-episode patients found that 87% responded to antipsychotic treatment within 12 months (Robinson et al 1999b). A number of other studies have shown that the early course of illness in schizophrenia and affective psychosis is turbulent and prone to relapse, with up to 80% of patients relapsing during the first 5 years (Robinson et al 1999a, Strakowski et al 1998, Vazquez-Barquero et al 1999, Wiersma et al 1998).

One of the most important considerations in the management of late recovery is the question of when to attempt cessation of antipsychotic medication, because long-term maintenance treatment is generally not recommended after a first episode of psychosis. A patient's level of vulnerability to further episodes of psychosis can be considered, based on factors such as premorbid functioning and personality, the duration and nature of their psychopathology, the level and stability of remission, and family history. Provision of continuing care is important (e.g. by a general practitioner) so that appropriate treatment can be initiated swiftly in the event of a recurrence of psychotic symptoms.

Medication should be continued for most, if not all, patients for at least 12 months after recovery from a first psychotic episode, and some authorities recommend that medication for a first episode of schizophrenia or schizoaffective disorder should continue for at least 2 years (Robinson et al 1999a). However,

it should be remembered that up to 25% of patients never relapse and some others will not relapse for many years. The timing of cessation of treatment will depend upon:

- the level of remission
- the duration of untreated psychosis
- whether persistent positive symptoms are present
- comorbid substance misuse
- ongoing stressful life circumstances
- level of functioning in a normal living situation

Patients should be aware that they are taking a calculated risk in stopping medication, and symptoms may return even when they have made a recovery. Patients may need to experience some return of symptoms to realize that a vulnerability to psychosis still exists, and that longer-term medication may be required. Clinical monitoring and a low threshold for reinstating medications should be considered, particularly in recent on-set schizophrenia (Gitlin et al 2001).

Withdrawal of medication should be tapered over some months and should only be stopped completely when stressful events in the patient's life are at minimal levels. If transient states of psychosis occur during the recovery period because of the presence of stressors (e.g. return to employment or school), then psychosocial support supplemented by an anxiolytic or mild tranquillizer may be adequate to contain the symptoms.

Other areas that can be addressed during the late recovery phase are the continuing vulnerability to psychosis (Nuechterlein et al 1992), the existence of comorbid or premorbid problems (such as anxiety disorders or sexual abuse) and the impact of these on the likelihood of relapse (Bermanzohn et al 2001).

Recovery tools

Psychoeducation

Psychoeducation is a core ingredient of case management and the 'building block' for most psychological interventions in early psychosis (see EPPIC 1997a, McGorry 1995b). Areas that should be covered by psychoeducation include:

- the nature of the illness
- the range of treatments that the person will be offered
- the patterns and variable nature of recovery
- prospects for the future
- agencies and personnel that will be involved in treatment

Local materials on first-episode psychosis that are suitable for patients and their families should be sought, or developed if they do not already exist. The capacity of patients and families to absorb information will vary depending on the circumstances of the illness, their background and level of education, and the presence or absence of factors such as denial or conflict. Some principles of psychoeducation are summarized in the text box.

Principles of psychoeducation
- Information should be introduced:
  - gradually
  - in digestible 'chunks'
  - when patients and families are psychologically ready to receive it
- Information may need to be repeated to enable reprocessing at a later stage in the course of the illness and its treatment. The level of understanding can be checked by asking people to retell their interpretation of the information that has been provided
- Information should be provided in a variety of media including video, recognizing that many people prefer formats other than conventional print-based booklets, pamphlets or information sheets
- Information alone might not produce the desired changes, as there may be psychological factors which act as barriers to change

Education materials used routinely at EPPIC are summarized in the text box and source details are provided in Appendix 1.

> **Psychoeducation materials routinely used with patient and families at EPPIC**
> - *Something is Not Quite Right* – pamphlet
> - *A Stitch in Time: Psychosis . . . Get Help Early* – community video
> - *A Stitch in Time: Psychosis . . . Get Help Early* – four information sheets
> - *The SANE Guide to Psychosis* – booklet
> - *Mood Swings and Mental Health* – booklet
> - *The Alice Guide to Psychosis* – interactive computer presentation
> - *Cannabis and Psychosis Fact Sheet*
> - *Trips and Journeys – Personal Accounts of Early Psychosis*
> - *Holding on to What is Real: A Video About Schizophrenia*
> - *Psychosis and Schizophrenia* – booklet
> - *Living with Schizophrenia: A Holistic Approach to Understanding, Preventing and Recovering from Negative Symptoms* – book
>
> See Appendix 1 for source details.

Cognitively Oriented Psychotherapy for Early Psychosis (COPE)

A brief cognitively-oriented psychotherapy, COPE has a focus on recovery from the first episode of psychosis. The goals of COPE are to promote adaptation to the experience of the illness and its treatment and to identify and reduce secondary morbidity (Jackson et al 1996, 1999, 2001a). Data from a COPE pilot study, using a non-randomized control group design, suggested that psychological benefits in the COPE group were generally sustained beyond the end of therapy (Jackson et al 1998, 2001b). A detailed account of the principles underlying the approach and practical guidelines for therapy can be found in the COPE manual (EPPIC 2001a).

Issues in recovery

Substance misuse

Substance misuse is one of the most common comorbid problems in first-episode psychosis (Hambrecht and Häfner 1996, Rabinowitz et al 1998, Strakowski et al 1995, 1996). It can be difficult to determine for any one individual whether substance misuse is an effect of the illness, whether it has contributed to the onset of psychosis, or both. On the one hand, substances may be abused as 'self-medication' in order to cope with distressing psychotic symptoms. On the other hand, the onset of psychosis may be precipitated in people who have other vulnerabilities to psychosis as a result of substance misuse. The EPPIC data suggest that approximately 70% of all first-episode patients have used illicit substances, predominantly cannabis, within 12 months prior to initial presentation for treatment (Power et al in press).

Substance misuse may lead to delays in accessing treatment, particularly if symptoms are attributed to substance misuse rather than an illness. Whatever the relationship between substance misuse and psychosis, it is associated with a poorer outcome (Kovasznay et al 1997, Linszen et al 1994).

The pattern of substance misuse is often variable in people with psychosis, and the emergence of psychotic symptoms can act as a powerful motivator to alter their drug habits. For example, the shock of experiencing a first episode of psychosis in association with heavy cannabis use is enough to lead to abstinence in some cases. If a person with psychosis attributes their illness to substance misuse, then it is appropriate to use this as a foundation for reinforcing a reduction in substance misuse.

There are several trends in current approaches to substance misuse which are applicable to people experiencing early psychosis (Edwards et al in press b):

- Brief interventions in people who attend health care services for other reasons are more effective then no intervention at all,

and may sometimes be as effective as more extensive treatment.

- Harm minimization may be a more realistic aim than abstinence. Harm from cannabis use can include exacerbation of psychosis, failure to respond to treatment and persistent illness, as well as financial, social and legal consequences.
- Treatment should be matched to an individual's readiness to change.
- A first psychotic episode can act as a powerful motivator to change, because the episode is often traumatic.

Intervention for cannabis use

A programme developed at EPPIC is investigating the value of a brief intervention for individuals with first-episode psychosis and 'problematic' cannabis use. The programme was prompted by difficulties in delivering effective interventions, for reasons including the following:

- separation of mental health services from drug and alcohol services in many cases
- lack of 'real world' guidance on interventions that are user-friendly, integrated within a comprehensive treatment programme, relevant, practical, individually tailored and able to be replicated
- lack of research

- a pervasive social view that cannabis is harmless
- individuals who use cannabis heavily being in a constant crisis which interferes with intervention

The programme recognizes that drug rehabilitation strategies are already delivered in a number of ways, including case management, group work, vocational rehabilitation, social skills training and accommodation support. However, many patients miss out on effective psychoeducation because of non-attendance or poor engagement or because there are inadequate resources to provide the service. The programme aims to develop an appreciation that cannabis use is potentially problematic in the context of any psychotic illness and to develop a commitment to change cannabis use. Ten sessions of one-to-one cognitive therapy are undertaken by clinical psychologists, based on psychoeducation about the effects of cannabis on psychosis and recovery and on motivational interviewing to obtain a commitment to change. A treatment manual is available (EPPIC 2002b).

Techniques for addressing the use of cannabis and other substances are outlined in the text box.

Techniques to address use of cannabis and other substances

- Make it clear that the use of the substance is detrimental for the individual – "you are one of the unlucky ones".
- Provide information about the links between psychosis and substance use.
- Explore reasons for substance use and develop alternative ways to provide these needs (e.g. relaxation, social contact).
- Concentrate on harm minimization – for example, avoid driving, avoid dangerous areas and activities, minimize the amounts used.
- Use the stages of change model – precontemplation precedes contemplation, which precedes action. The process of change may take time.
- Recruit peers to discourage substance use.

Prolonged recovery

Poor response to treatment may be associated with a longer duration of untreated psychosis and the total period of active psychosis. Early identification and specialized treatment of patients who do not achieve rapid remission after their first psychotic episode has the potential to accelerate the recovery process and change the course of the disorder. For some patients it may be possible to prevent the establishment of treatment resistance.

Failure to recover can result from a number of reasons including non-adherence to treatment, depression, concurrent substance misuse, lack of responsiveness to medication and the patient's environment (including the family situation). It can manifest in several ways, including:

- persistence of positive symptoms
- presence of negative symptoms
- enduring affective disturbance

Principles of treatment of positive symptoms include:

- active pursuit of effective treatment, commencing with relatively low-dose strategies but being prepared to increase the dose modestly or change the antipsychotic medication if response is delayed beyond 6 weeks
- an expectation that at least two adequate antipsychotic medication trials within a 3-month period may be needed (with 'adequacy' based on doses equivalent to haloperidol 10 mg)
- use of atypical antipsychotics such as risperidone and olanzapine as 'first-line' treatments

- augmentation with lithium over a 4- to 6-week period if appropriate (Kane and Marder 1993)
- the early introduction of clozapine if required (Kane and Marder 1993, Lieberman 1996, Meltzer 1995)
- use of strategies to promote treatment compliance, including psychoeducation
- early addition of structured psychological and family approaches
- attention to substance misuse
- conveying hope to the patient and family, but acknowledging that recovery will take longer for some people.

Prolonged recovery – TREAT/STOPP

- The Treatment Resistance Early Assessment Team (TREAT) at EPPIC identifies individuals who are experiencing persisting positive and/or negative symptoms following their first or subsequent acute episode (Edwards et al in press c). It provides a consultancy service to EPPIC case managers and doctors, aiming to accelerate recovery and prevent established treatment resistance. The Systematic Treatment of Persistent Positive Symptoms (STOPP) programme was developed to help treat enduring positive psychotic symptoms (Edwards et al 1998, Herrmann-Doig et al in press). A manual detailing the TREAT approach is available (EPPIC 2001d).

A randomized controlled trial is being conducted to establish the effectiveness of the early introduction of STOPP and the use of clozapine. Consecutive first-episode patients not achieving a predefined level of remission after the initial 12 weeks of treatment are randomized into one of four groups for a further 12-week period: thioridazine, thioridazine and STOPP, clozapine, or clozapine and STOPP.

Suicide prevention

Some patients with psychiatric illness are at high risk of suicide and require specific attention to suicide risk during recovery (Kulkarni and Power 1999). For example, one in five young men with adolescent-onset schizophrenia commits suicide (Krausz et al 1995), and patients are at highest risk of suicide during the early postpsychotic period (Drake et al 1984). In addition, substance misuse disorders are evident in 30–70% of youth suicide victims, either alone or in conjunction with other major psychiatric disorders (Shafii et al 1988).

No strategies have been shown conclusively to be effective in preventing suicide, but some data suggest the following interventions may be helpful:

- Psychological interventions: cognitive–behavioural therapy interventions such as COPE (see page 53) may reduce the risk of suicide indirectly through effects on the primary and secondary symptoms of psychosis and on adaptation.
- Psychosocial interventions include intensive support during the early recovery phase and psychoeducation.
- Possible pharmacological interventions include the following:
  - Trials of the newer antipsychotics have shown promising results, having fewer side effects and perhaps a greater effect on negative symptoms and cognition than conventional antipsychotics.
  - Early use of clozapine in treatment-resistant psychosis may reduce the risk of suicide (Meltzer and Okayli 1995).
  - Combined use of antipsychotics and antidepressants or electroconvulsive therapy (ECT) in acute depressive psychosis may be beneficial (Parker et al 1992, Rothschild et al 1993, Spiker

et al 1985). The use of antidepressants with antipsychotics appears to be beneficial in patients with postpsychotic depression (Siris et al 1994).

LifeSPAN suicide prevention programme

LifeSPAN is a cognitive–behavioural therapy intervention directed towards feelings of hopelessness, suicidal ideation and depression. It was specifically tailored for patients with first-episode psychosis, to be used in consultation with suicide experts (Power 1999). The programme detects and treats patients who attend EPPIC and are judged to be at very high risk of suicide. Results of a randomized controlled trial suggested that cognitive indicators of suicide risk, such as hopelessness, 'reasons for living' and suicidal ideation, improved significantly more in the group receiving LifeSPAN compared to the group receiving standard clinical care (Power et al 1999). A LifeSPAN treatment manual details the approach (EPPIC 2002d).

Personality difficulties

The interaction between personality and functional psychoses is complex, particularly in patients with first-episode psychosis (Hulbert et al 1996). These patients are usually young and might not have fully developed their personality and sense of self. Treatment difficulties that may relate to a 'personality disorder' require specific investigation. Possible relationships between personality and psychosis include:

- a disturbance in behaviour occurring as an attenuated form of psychotic disorder
- personality traits acting as a predisposing factor for a psychotic disorder
- personality changes occurring as a complication of psychosis
- personality traits acting as risk factors for relapse
- the presence of comorbid personality disorder

It is important to be aware that patient's personality may influence the expression of illness, and that the illness will influence their personality function.

EPPIC service developments

Outpatient case management

Two multidisciplinary teams at EPPIC provide case management and medical treatment based on geographical boundaries of the service's catchment area. Inpatient and outpatient treatment revolves around the clinician–patient relationship. Goals of case management include (Edwards et al 1999):

- minimizing the duration of active psychosis
- supporting medication strategies for first-episode psychosis
- providing acute treatment in collaboration with the YAT and/or the inpatient team
- providing psychoeducation to patients and families
- actively seeking and treating secondary problems

Elements of COPE are incorporated within the outpatient case management service.

With a steady case load of about 400 patients, EPPIC has an average of 22 new cases accepted every month. Full-time case managers carry case loads of about 30 patients, and each patient is also assigned a psychiatrist or senior psychiatry registrar. Case allocation and case loads are carefully and systematically monitored. The frequency of clinician–patient contact varies with the phase of illness and the patient's involvement with other programmes. All patients are reviewed regularly by the outpatient team throughout a standard 18-month follow-up period. A handbook provides details of the approach to case management (EPPIC 2001a).

Family work

Family interventions at EPPIC focus on three elements (Gleeson et al 1999):

- the impact of the illness on the family system
- the impact of the illness on individual family members
- the interaction between the family and the course of the psychosis

Assessment of the family situation includes identifying their explanatory models for the psychosis, cultural issues and religious beliefs. The needs of families for crisis support and practical education about psychosis are addressed through multi-family group interventions and individual sessions with families, supported by specialist family workers. An integrated approach incorporates psychoeducation, crisis management, practical problem solving, supportive psychotherapy and, if indicated, family therapy. Psychoeducation includes a series of evening sessions entitled 'Family and Friends' scheduled over 4 consecutive weeks, covering aspects of psychosis, treatment approaches and the future. These sessions have also been condensed and run as a single 'workshop' in Greek and Vietnamese, and there are plans for presentations in Italian, Croatian, Arabic and Turkish.

As a component of the TREAT clinic (see

pages 56–57), a second multi-family intervention provides support and psychoeducation for families that have a relative who has more persistent illness. The group meets for about 90 minutes fortnightly for 6 months. Topics include promoting a positive emotional environment and emotional issues such as grief and loss. A manual on family work is available (EPPIC 1997b). A support group for siblings is also offered.

Social treatments

The EPPIC group programme provides a range of groups focused on the acute and recovery phases of illness. The acute group programme in the inpatient unit is activity-oriented and reality-based, and it aims to provide structure, decrease the trauma of admission and assist recovery. The recovery group programme operates on four 10-week cycles each year and caters for approximately 50 clients each cycle. Participants select groups to assist with achieving their personal goals, identified in collaboration with group programme staff. Groups encompass five streams:

- social/recreational
- vocational/educational
- health promotion
- creative expression
- personal development

Evaluation data suggest the group programme attracts individuals with poorer premorbid adjustment and that attendance may assist in preventing deterioration and disability (Albiston et al 1998). A manual on the group programme provides details of the approach (EPPIC 2000b).

Vocational rehabilitation

The outpatient case manager coordinates the delivery of vocational rehabilitation through a brokerage system. The group programme has a specialist vocational stream that incorporates prevocational skill development and vocational planning. Consultation with occupational therapists is available for assessment and planning. Teachers are available on-site to work individually with 15- to 18-year old patients on aspects of school, training or employment (about one-third of patients in this age group are not involved in any substantial work, study or training activity).

There is a diverse network of government and non-government community-based services available to support vocational rehabilitation. Mainstream educational and employment services are used where possible, as they are likely to have a normalizing influence. However, specialist psychiatric vocational services are often used as stepping stones to mainstream services. A regular forum is held for clinicians and providers of vocational services to ensure good communication between the participants.

Accommodation

Through a collaborative accommodation project with the Schizophrenia Fellowship of Victoria, EPPIC has access to four self-contained 1-bed units for young people who are homeless or at risk of homelessness.

Community support workers attached to each unit assist with issues such as problem solving, time management, organization of leisure time, living skills, identification of alternative long-term housing, and continuing assessment of the person's progress through the recovery phase. This medium-term housing option assumes that the majority of young people will recover from psychosis and then move into mainstream housing.

Multi-component early intervention – models of good practice

5

Given the limited number of studies conducted thus far to investigate the benefits and challenges of early intervention, there is a need to establish clinical and research centres for this purpose. (Malla and Norman 1999, p. 396)

Assessing the impact of early detection and prevention programs requires a co-ordinated catchment-based health service. (Fenton 1997, p. 43)

Overview

The 1990s saw a rapid expansion of early psychosis initiatives (Edwards et al 2000). Developments in western countries include the following:

- Australia and New Zealand have an active approach to early intervention, which includes the establishment of networks and interest groups, attempts to influence health policy, and strong and diverse service initiatives. Interest has been fuelled by early psychosis conferences held in Australia at national (1994, 1998) and international levels.

Table 5.1
Multi-element models

	Year commenced	Diagnosis	Intake age (years)	Follow-up period (years	Services provided
Early Psychosis Prevention and Intervention Centre (EPPIC), Melbourne	1992 (inpatient unit since 1984)	FEP	15–29	1.5	Inpatient Outpatient Prodrome
Early Treatment and Identification of Psychosis (TIPS) project, Norway and Denmark	1997	Schizophrenia spectrum and affective disorders with incongruent delusions/hallucinations	18–65	2	Outpatient Prodrome
Early Intervention Service (EIS), Birmingham, UK	1995	FEP	16–30	3	Outpatient Prodrome
Early Psychosis Program (EPP), Calgary, Alberta, Canada	1996	Non-affective FEP	16–45	3	Outpatient Prodrome
Prevention and Early Intervention Program for Psychosis (PEPP), London, Ontario, Canada	1996	Non-affective FEP	16–50	2	Inpatient Outpatient

FEP, First-episode psychosis

- Early psychosis initiatives are widespread in Europe, with considerable activities under way in Scandinavia, German-speaking countries and The Netherlands.

Attempts to systematize the early psychosis focus are progressing in the UK through major policy reform (Lewis and Drake 2001) and this is likely to have a

Catchment area population	New cases per year	Estimated standing case load	Evaluation	Funding	Contact
819 000 206 279 in 15–29 age range	255 (average 1997–2000)	400+	Process; impact; outcome at 6, 12, 24 months for subsamples	Recurrent	www.eppic.org.au
370 000 (Rogaland) 190 000 (Oslo) 95 000 (Roskilde)	100	n/a	Outcome at 3 months, 1, 2 and 5 years; intervention group compared with 2 non-intervention groups	6-Year project (1997–2002)	www.tips-info.com
300 000 (1 million from 3/2002)	120	150	Outcome at 1, 2 and 3 years	Recurrent	www.iris-initiative.org.uk m.j.birchwood.20@bham.ac.uk fax: 0044 121 685 6049
930 000 (city of Calgary	85	170	Outcome at 3, 6, 9, 12, 15, 18, 21, 24 months, and 3 years	Recurrent	www.early-psychosis.com
390 000 (London and Middlesex)	50	100	Outcome at 1 and 2 years	Recurrent	www.pepp.ca akmalla@julian.uwo.ca Terry.McLean@lhsc.on.ca

significant impact on the national efforts of neighbouring countries. Interest is developing in Italy, Spain, Portugal and France.

- North American services have contributed significantly to the momentum with substantial activity in early psychosis research and, more recently, development of pilot clinical programmes. Several key services have been established in the USA (see Chapter 8). Canada is taking a leading role in early psychosis, with developments in most provinces.

Early psychosis service initiatives are also developing in other parts of the world. Major projects are under way in Hong Kong and Singapore, and there has been interest shown in Japan, China, Indonesia, Cambodia and Pakistan. A first-episode clinic has been established in Cape Town, South Africa, and an early psychosis interest group is being considered in Brazil.

This chapter describes five well-advanced multi-element models of early intervention which focus on early detection *and* provision of optimal treatment, and are engaged in substantial clinical research. Table 5.1 provides 'facts and figures' regarding these five models, which need to be examined in conjunction with the text. Many other quality programmes exist, and these five examples have been selected to exemplify the issues involved.

In each case, the model is briefly described and guidance provided on how to obtain further information. National and international collaborative links with other programmes, in terms of research and service delivery, are also described. Each of the services readily share their knowledge and resource materials.

Early Psychosis Prevention and Intervention Centre (EPPIC), Melbourne, Victoria, Australia

The early psychosis initiative now known as EPPIC has evolved steadily since 1984 (Edwards et al 1994, Edwards and McGorry 1998, McGorry et al 1996). The programme began with a specialized inpatient ward for first-episode cases, located in the grounds of a major psychiatric hospital serving the inner-city area of Melbourne (Copolov et al 1989). Experience with first-episode psychosis led to increased recognition of the special needs of patients and the limitations of a programme restricted to inpatient care.

The EPPIC model aims to reduce the level of both primary and secondary morbidity in patients with early psychosis, through the dual strategy of identifying patients as early as possible after the onset of illness and providing intensive phase-specific treatment for up to 18 months.

The EPPIC catchment area covers the western metropolitan region of Melbourne, an area served by four geographically based adult mental health services. Important features of the region include a high proportion of people born in other countries or with at least one parent born in another country, many people with a low fluency in English, low income, high unemployment, and a low proportion of people with university qualifications. Fewer

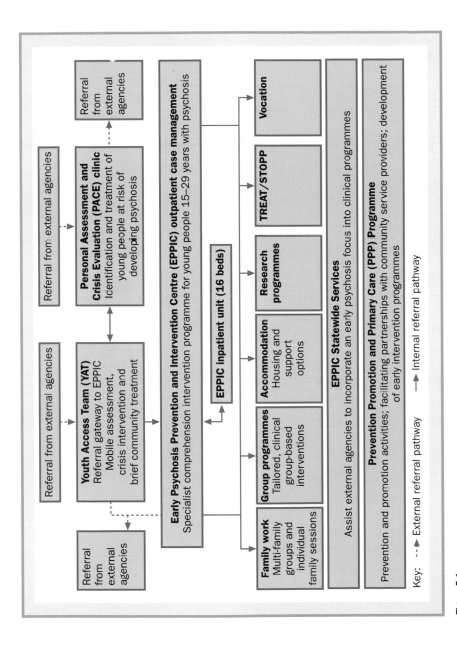

Figure 5.1
The EPPIC service model c.2001.

than 20 private psychiatrists serve the catchment area.

The service components of EPPIC, which are illustrated in Figure 5.1, include:

- a mobile assessment and treatment team (YAT) (see Chapter 2)
- prevention, promotion and primary care activities (for example the Compass Project and the General Practitioner Associate Programme – see Chapter 2)
- a prodrome clinic (PACE – see Chapter 2)
- a 16-bed inpatient unit (see Chapter 3)
- outpatient case management (see Chapter 4)
- family work (see Chapter 4)
- a group programme (see Chapter 4)
- prolonged recovery clinics (TREAT/STOPP – see Chapter 4).

There is also access to an intensive mobile outreach service for youths who are difficult to engage in treatment.

Structures to facilitate admission of the young people and their families into the EPPIC programme are in place (see text box).

> **Input of patients and families**
> The **Platform Project** provides an environment that supports, advocates, responds to and sustains active participation by young people in EPPIC activities. A group of eight current or former patients, who are paid for their input, meet monthly with some guidance from programme staff. The 'Platform Team' acts as an advocacy body and produces a bimonthly newsletter.
>
> The **Family Participation Project** establishes a range of avenues for family members, partners and friends of EPPIC patients to provide feedback to the service (including expressing views at management level), attend support groups to assist other families, and develop volunteer training programmes and paid positions for family members. A structure that allows families of new clients to access support from families of current or discharged patients has also been established.

There are 60 equivalent full-time clinical staff positions at EPPIC and another 30 staff employed in research, special projects and education. An evaluation and quality officer assesses the impact of EPPIC programmes (see Chapter 7). Operational details, including the organizational structure, working group committee structures, staff development and supervision arrangements are contained in the *Youth Pack* (EPPIC 2001b), which is reviewed twice yearly. The *Youth Pack* also contains information on the broader youth mental health programme in which the EPPIC service is embedded.

Research activities include the duration of

untreated psychosis, prolonged recovery, use of cannabis and nicotine, cognitively oriented psychotherapies, suicide prevention, impact of personality on psychosis, emotion recognition, psychopharmacology and adjunctive medication strategies for schizophrenia-related disorders, role of potentially neuropathogenic infectious agents, relapse, treatment adherence strategies, neuroimaging, neurocognition, neuroendocrine studies, and the prediction and prevention of transition to psychoses.

Evaluation of EPPIC – the 1996 paper and current projects

A naturalistic effectiveness study was undertaken to evaluate the EPPIC programme, comparing 12-month outcomes among 51 patients treated under the EPPIC model in 1993 with a historical cohort of 51 patients with first-episode psychosis from the same catchment area treated under the previous generic model of care between 1989 and 1992 (McGorry et al 1996). The EPPIC patients experienced a significantly better outcome than their counterparts with regard to overall quality of life, including social and role functioning. The level of post-traumatic stress associated with hospitalization and other elements of treatment was reduced, and the experience of

psychosis itself was less traumatic. The average length of hospital stay and the mean dose of antipsychotic medication both decreased, without compromising recovery. The mean duration of untreated psychosis was reduced from 237 to 191 days, but the difference was not statistically significant. Improved short-term outcomes were likely to result from improvements in phase-specific treatment and intensity of treatment, rather than the earlier provision of treatment. The increased costs of providing more intensive community-based care were more than compensated by the reduction in inpatient care costs (Mihalopoulos et al 1999). A further study suggested that only patients with a mid-range duration of untreated psychosis (1–6 months) experienced significantly better outcomes than patients treated in the previous model of care (Carbone et al 1999).

Evaluation projects in progress include comparison of an EPPIC cohort with concurrent cohorts of first-episode psychosis patients from two other Melbourne catchment areas (Krstev et al 2001b) and medium-term follow up of 200 pre-EPPIC patients and 145 EPPIC patients described by McGorry et al (1996). Planned evaluations include the extent of adherence to clinical practice guidelines, and a randomized controlled trial of the total EPPIC treatment package delivered over a 3-year period of care.

Relationship with state-wide mental health services

Since 1995 EPPIC has aimed to ensure all mental health agencies in the State of Victoria (population about 5 million) have access to clinical skills, expertise and knowledge in early psychosis. Statewide Services (a subprogramme of EPPIC) provides:

- secondary and tertiary consultation
- professional education and training
- resource development
- *Early Psychosis Projects* (1996–2000), which develop models of practice responsive to local needs and service structures in discrete regions (see Chapter 8)
- support to a state network of 18 early psychosis workers

National Early Psychosis Project

The Australian health system is based on a complex mix of funding and service provision

by the federal government (the Government of the Commonwealth of Australia) and the governments of six states and two territories. The *National Mental Health Strategy* (www.health.gov.au/hsdd/mentalhe/resources/index.htm), a joint initiative of the federal and State/Territory governments, commissioned the National Early Psychosis Project (NEPP), which commenced in 1996 and continued until January 1998 (Pennell and McGorry 2001). The NEPP was managed by EPPIC and aimed to develop and promote a national model of best practice for early intervention in psychosis. The NEPP had three foci:

- professional education and training
- service and policy development
- information dissemination.

Eight state and territory coordinators progressed the project in conjunction with government health departments, mental health professionals, young people and their families, and other stakeholders. A model of contextual factors in implementing best practice treatment in early psychosis was developed, outlined in Figure 5.2. The project resulted in a high level of education and training activities across all states and territories (Joyce and Hurworth 1998):

- Multiple early psychosis projects are in operation in each of the five most

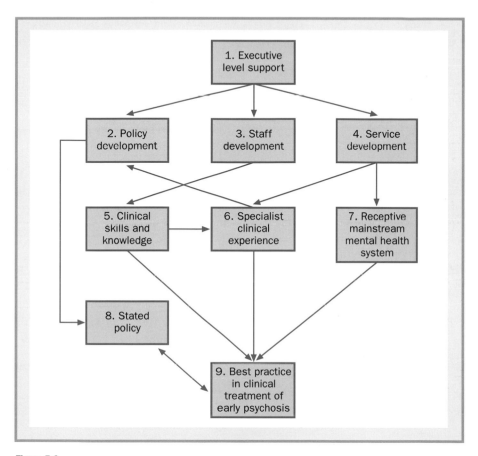

Figure 5.2
Contextual factors affecting the implementation of best practice treatment in early psychosis in mental health settings.
Adapted with permission of Centre for Program Evaluation, from Joyce C, Hurworth R (1998) Evaluation of the National Early Psychosis Project: Final Report. *Melbourne: Centre for Program Evaluation, University of Melbourne.*

populated states. New South Wales, with a population of about 8 million, has 36 such projects (New South Wales Health Department 2000a).

- Networks were developed, such as the Early Psychosis Group in Perth, Western Australia, which continues to hold regular meetings to develop knowledge and skills.

- A training video, *Getting in Early: Sally's Story* (1998) was produced, presenting a 'hypothetical' on pathways to care and panel discussion.
- The Australian Clinical Guidelines for Early Psychosis (National Early Psychosis Project Clinical Guidelines Working Party 1998) were developed (see Appendix 2). The Commonwealth Government subsequently initiated a tender for evaluation of their implementation.
- Policy is most advanced in New South Wales (New South Wales Health Department 2000b) and there are plans in place to advance national policy further.
- The third Australian Early Psychosis Conference was held in October 2001.

Early Intervention Service (EIS), Birmingham, UK

The EIS in Birmingham, UK, commenced at the Archer Centre in 1990. Evolving from a psychosocial programme within a large state psychiatric hospital, EIS focused on young people, including many with established psychosis. Since 1995 EIS has developed into a service exclusively for people experiencing first-episode psychosis (Jackson and Farmer 1998, Spencer et al 2001). The aims of the service are to:

- reduce the duration of untreated psychosis
- accelerate remission

- reduce adverse personal reactions and maximize social and work functioning
- prevent relapse and treatment resistance
- sustain engagement within a single service over a 3-year period

The EIS is part of the Northern Birmingham Mental Health National Health Service Trust, which also includes 24-hour psychiatric emergency and home treatment teams, primary care and liaison services, assertive outreach, and rehabilitation and recovery services. It covers an inner-city multi-ethnic catchment area with a high psychiatric morbidity. About 30% of EIS patients are African-Caribbean and 30% Asian. The EIS is due to expand its services across the city of Birmingham to a total catchment area of 1 million. The service will provide support and assistance in national developments in conjunction with the Initiative to Reduce the Impact of Schizophrenia (IRIS – see page 74).

The EIS intake team screens and assesses new referrals, and each client is assigned a key worker who is responsible for the coordination of care. The core component of EIS is an assertive outreach team, operating 7 days per week and staffed by 10 case managers (mostly psychiatric nurses) with case loads of 15 individuals. Key workers are trained in identifying early warning signs of relapse and in behavioural family therapy. Other professionals, such as psychologists and occupational therapists, assist in the delivery of interventions that follow agreed protocols and include:

- low-dose antipsychotic regimes
- cognitive therapy for delusions and hallucinations
- cognitive therapy aimed at improving adjustment and reducing comorbidity
- psychosocial intervention for problem drug and alcohol use
- prevocational training

Former service users are employed as support workers in the outreach team and respite units. A family and carers' support group meets monthly. Patients are represented on the management group and on all interview panels, and there is a 'consumer forum' and newsletter. Input by consumers is encouraged and complaints are dealt with personally by the director.

Individuals requiring acute care are admitted to the adult psychiatric facility and visited daily by the case manager. There is a residential/respite facility based in a nearby house which caters for up to four individuals who require more intensive input because of prolonged recovery time or who cannot be managed in the community.

Outcomes such as duration of untreated psychosis, pathways to care, symptoms, relapse and quality of life are assessed and used to refine service delivery. Staff meet weekly for supervision and training, providing a forum for discussion of difficult cases, monitoring standards of care and resource development. Examination of early outcome data suggests that EIS has promoted engagement and reduced suicide rates.

As one of five centres participating in a European Commission joint research venture on medicosocial health care systems (see text box), EIS is involved in developing a prodrome clinic.

European Prediction of Psychosis Study

The European Prediction of Psychosis Study (EPOS) is a collaborative multicentre study with participating centres in the UK, Spain, Finland, Germany and The Netherlands. As indicated by the title, the major focus of EPOS is to predict the transition from prodrome to psychosis. The objectives are to:

- describe and compare pathways to care for persons at risk of psychosis
- provide a systematic multi-level assessment of indicators for the risk of psychosis
- evaluate the predictive validity of these variables
- assess disabilities in prodromal states

- achieve preliminary development and description of therapeutic and preventive interventions

Designed as a prospective longitudinal field study, EPOS has repeated measures at nine and 18 months to monitor the individuals at risk and examine how they gain access to, and receive treatment from, a specialized health care system. At least 50 prodromal individuals are expected to be recruited by each centre. The consortium is managed centrally by a coordinating centre based in Cologne, supported by a steering group and an international advisory board. The study is funded by the European Commission.

Enquiries:
heinrich.reventlow@medizin.uni-koeln.de

Initiative to Reduce the Impact of Schizophrenia (IRIS)

The EIS has been a driving force behind a West Midlands initiative known as IRIS, created in 1996 as a response to concerns about services for young people with psychosis (www.iris-initiative.org.uk). The initiative aims to promote early intervention and improve partnerships between primary and secondary care (Macmillan and Shiers 2000). Standards of care drafted by the group aim to achieve:

- early detection and initiation of therapy
- low-dose antipsychotic therapy and use of benzodiazepines during the acute phase
- cognitive therapy to promote recovery from psychosis and trauma
- facilitated access to training/employment
- family support
- relapse prevention
- use of home treatment where possible.

The network of services across the West Midlands linked to IRIS have been awarded status as a 'Beacon' service (a government-sponsored mechanism to identify services offering good practice and coordinate dissemination of expertise) with resources for site visits, placements, training and mentoring arrangements. The Department of Health commissioned IRIS to produce *Early Intervention in Psychosis: Clinical Guidelines and Service Frameworks and Tool Kit*, (www.iris-initiative.org.uk) to support early psychosis initiatives.

National plan

In July 2000 the UK government announced an unprecedented 33% rise in health care spending over the next 3 years (*The NHS Plan*, www.nhs.uk/national plan/nhsplan.htm). Mental health was nominated as one of three priority areas. The government's blueprint for mental health services included dedicated home treatment, assertive outreach and early intervention in psychosis. The plan stated that:

> *Early intervention to reduce the period of untreated psychosis in young people can prevent initial problems, and improve long-term outcomes:*
>
> - *fifty early intervention teams will be established over the next three years to provide treatment and active support in the community to these young people and their families*
> - *by 2004 all young people who experience a first episode of psychosis, such as schizophrenia, will receive the early and intensive support they need. This will benefit 7,500 young people each year.* (p. 119).

This ambitious strategy was influenced by lobbying and promotion of the early intervention paradigm by IRIS and the National Schizophrenia Fellowship. Arguments were advanced to the government on four levels:

- the poor quality of existing services and

confused access points for young people experiencing psychosis for the first time
- the need for services to be youth-friendly and sustained
- the need to improve access to training and employment
- early intervention may forestall secondary problems such as school drop out, unemployment, forensic issues, and self-harm or suicide

The concept of early intervention as a secondary prevention strategy was not advanced as the principal argument, recognizing the fact that a number of key strategies were incomplete. This strategy circumvented potential objections about 'lack of evidence' (see Chapter 8).

The commissioning framework, published by the Department of Health in March 2001 as part of its *Mental Health Policy Implementation Guide* (www.doh.gov.uk/mentalhealth/implementationguide.htm), was launched at a conference in Birmingham, to which the Minister of Health invited all Health Authority and Mental Health Trust Chief Executives and Directors of Social Services. Fifty teams, located in 126 local implementation areas, will target 14- to 35-year-olds, and each will accept about 150 new cases per year. Treatment will be provided for the first 3 years of illness, leading to total loads of 450 cases of first-episode psychosis per team. Based on EIS, the teams will provide:

- an assertive team model with a case load ratio of 1:15
- comprehensive support and engagement for 3 years through the 'critical period' following onset of psychosis
- home treatment and exclusive access to dedicated community-based respite units
- service users and youth workers employed as support staff
- a focus on employment
- a strategy to reduce untreated psychosis through collaboration with primary care and community agencies.

Early Treatment and Identification of Psychosis (TIPS), Norway and Denmark

During the early 1980s there was a reorganization of psychiatric services in Rogaland county, situated on the south-west coast of Norway, with a gradual closing of the state psychiatric hospital. These changes were accompanied by an interest in establishing more systematic treatments for early schizophrenia, and it was decided to give priority to first-episode cases. 'Schizophrenia Days', an annual week-long conference about psychosis for professionals and the public, was initiated in 1989.

In 1993–1994 a pilot study on duration of untreated psychosis was undertaken in the region. It identified long delays in detection (mean 114 weeks, median 26 weeks), and a

longer duration of untreated psychosis was correlated with poorer outcome (Larsen et al 1999, 2000, in press). The findings strengthened the resolve to establish health service programmes for early detection and treatment of schizophrenia (Johannessen et al 2000).

A prospective, longitudinal 5-year study, TIPS aims to investigate whether early identification and optimal treatment of first-episode psychosis leads to better outcomes (Larsen et al 2000a, Johannessen et al 1999, 2000, 2001, in press). Research support and collaboration occurs through the University of Oslo in Sweden and Yale University in the USA. The design is quasi-experimental (the research team considered it unethical to randomize patients to control conditions such as a long waiting list with no treatment): It will compare first-episode patients at three sites. A site in Rogaland county will continue its focus on early detection, while control sites in Ullevål sector (Oslo) and Roskilde (Denmark) will continue with usual practice. Information on a historical control group treated previously in Rogaland (no early detection, no treatment protocol) is also being examined.

The trial programme includes:

- extensive public education on the early signs of psychosis
- specific education for teachers, youth and general practitioners

- clinical teams with a primary responsibility for early detection of individuals with untreated first-episode psychosis

A treatment protocol is based mainly on the Schizophrenia Patient Outcome Team (PORT) treatment recommendations (Lehman et al 1998). The protocol was derived by consensus among a number of medical directors of psychosis services and is used at all sites over a 2-year period, applied within the usual treatment framework. The protocol includes:

- weekly supportive 'flexible psychotherapy' (Fenton 2000) by psychodynamic psychotherapists with active outreach
- a standard low-dose medication regimen, commencing with olanzapine then switching if necessary to risperidone, then perphenazine, and finally clozapine
- family work (individual family sessions, family workshop, and biweekly family sessions) focusing on problem solving and psychoeducation (McFarlane 2000, in press)

The protocol specifies different non-pharmacological therapy and duration of maintenance medication for different diagnoses (for details see the protocol, available in English, at www.tips-info.com). Inpatients are admitted to general psychiatric units. In the first year of the study

(1997–1998 cohort) the modal number of admissions was one and the median length of inpatient stay was 13 weeks. The psychotherapist acts as case manager and receives monthly group supervision.

Evaluation of patients occurs at baseline, 3 months, and 1, 2 and 5 years. Treatment packages are reviewed for each patient at 1- and 2-year follow ups. Assessment includes diagnosis, premorbid functioning, duration of prodromal symptoms and untreated psychosis, level of symptoms, social interaction, quality of life and global functioning, deficit symptoms, drug and alcohol use, life events, expressed emotion and cognitive function.

The Rogaland county early detection team received recurrent funding which will allow the detection service to continue beyond the life of the research project.

The TIPS Project – positive early data on duration of untreated psychosis

Preliminary data indicate that duration of untreated psychosis has been significantly reduced in Rogaland ($n = 32$, mean 17 weeks, median 12 weeks) compared with the historical controls ($n = 43$, mean 2.1 years, median 26 weeks). Similarly, early data from the 1997–1998 cohort show a significantly shorter duration of untreated psychosis in Rogaland ($n = 67$, mean 24 weeks, median 4 weeks) compared with Oslo/Roskilde ($n = 68$, mean 60 weeks, median 12 weeks). The figures suggest that the information campaigns have been effective in assisting early detection (Larsen et al, 2001b).

National implementation

A national implementation conference on early intervention for Norwegian county medical officers was held during 2001. Early psychosis initiatives are in progress in the cities of Telemark, Bergen, Akershus and Nordland.

Prevention and Early Intervention Program for Psychoses (PEPP), London, Ontario, Canada

The objectives of PEPP are to:

*   provide comprehensive assessment and treatment for individuals with a non-affective first episode of psychosis
*   promote early diagnosis and intervention strategies
*   conduct research on the early phases of psychosis, including the impact of early intervention

The programme includes an outpatient service and accesses a 16-bed psychosis inpatient unit (which rarely houses more than four to six PEPP patients). Treatment is based on a stress-vulnerability model for the development and course of psychotic disorders (Nuechterlein and Dawson 1984, Norman and Malla 1993) and follows a protocol combining optimum pharmacological and psychosocial interventions.

Screening is provided within 24–48 hours of referral and, if psychosis is indicated, a full assessment is undertaken within 1 week depending on the urgency of the referral. A large-scale community case detection initiative is in progress, using brochures, posters, a calendar, bookmarks in student admission packages, local radio, community fund-raising events and a 30-second television commercial on early signs of psychosis. Consumers have been involved in planning, fundraising and the dissemination of case detection material to the community. Individuals considered to be 'at risk for psychosis' receive an open trial of supportive therapy, including stress management and problem solving with regular review, although a formal prodrome clinic is not in operation.

The outpatient service uses assertive clinical case management in which psychiatrists, psychologists and occupational therapists provide specific treatments, but the primary responsibility for patient care lies with the nurse/social worker case manager.

Atypical antipsychotics are preferred. Clozapine is offered if patients do not respond adequately to at least two other atypical antipsychotics, or if there has been little or no response after 12 months. Group interventions are designed to facilitate transition from the acute stage to stabilization; support groups and cognitive skills training are also provided. Individual cognitive–behavioural therapy aimed at comorbidity, psychotic symptoms and self-worth is available from a psychologist by referral.

The family intervention consists of two primary components: a series of three 2-hour psychoeducational workshops delivered 3 weeks apart and repeated throughout the year, and individual family work provided by the social worker, case manager and psychiatrist. A multiple family group has been established for patients who continue to have problems beyond the first 2 years. Families are also encouraged to participate in the self-help parent support group established by parents of first-episode patients (see Chapter 8). A series of three 25- to 35-minute teaching videos and a workbook have been developed for families (PEPP 2000b). These are designed for initial use with the assistance of a clinician, and then for families to use on their own or for discussion purposes in support groups.

At the end of the 2-year programme most patients are transferred to 'medical management' and continue to seen by their psychiatrists within the programme. About 15% are deemed to be in need of ongoing case management and they continue in the full programme for an additional year.

Screening, assessment and treatment manuals detail the approach (PEPP 2000a, www.pepp.ca). The service is staffed by 15 clinicians who work across inpatient and community components, up to five inpatient nurses, and nine full-time research staff in addition to research faculty members.

Quality of life of PEPP patients
Data are available from a representative community sample of 41 PEPP patients at baseline assessment, after clinical stabilization and 1 year later (Malla et al 2001a). There were highly significant improvements in most dimensions of self-reported quality of life which were generally independent of changes in symptoms. The results provide support for the conclusion that comprehensive phase-specific treatment beyond symptom remission has a positive impact in schizophrenia spectrum disorders.

Ontario provincial government

An Ontario Working Group on Early Intervention in Psychosis has been established for promoting early intervention within the province (www.cmha.ca). The group is committed to bringing the benefits of early treatment to all citizens of Ontario who experience the onset of psychosis, and to their families. The government has funded a 1-year study in four sites to set up a database and track patient outcomes in terms of symptoms, quality of life and service satisfaction; PEPP will operate as the coordinating centre for the study.

National initiative

In 1999 PEPP obtained a Canadian federal government research grant to assist in establishing a consortium of early intervention research programmes. This is now part of the Canadian Institutes of Health Research (CIHR). Consortium grants are designed to allow a group of researchers working in a new area to develop a research agenda. The Early Psychosis Consortium has reviewed potential areas of collaboration and submitted a report to CIHR.

Early Psychosis Program (EPP), Calgary, Alberta, Canada

The EPP, funded by a competitive grant from the Alberta Provincial Mental Health Advisory Board, provides a comprehensive 3-year service to individuals experiencing non-

affective first-episode psychosis (Addington and Addington 2001a). Treatment comprises:

- assignment of a psychiatrist and case manager who undertake assessment, monitoring, pharmacotherapy and supportive therapy
- cognitive therapy to help adaptation to the psychotic illness, address secondary morbidity and reduce psychotic symptoms
- groups such as 'Psychosis Education', 'Recovery Group', 'Moving on Group', 'Good Health Modules' and 'Substance Use' (Addington and Addington 2001b)
- individual family work over six to eight sessions in the first year, focusing on education about psychosis, recommendations for coping with the disorder, communication skills and problem solving training, followed by a six-session multi-family group (Addington et al in press)
- continued assessment, case management and family work during inpatient admission to any of three city hospitals

Ongoing evaluation includes symptoms, side effects, quality of life, substance use, social functioning, neurocognition and effect on the family. During the first 4 years of operation, 395 referrals were received and 284 individuals were engaged in treatment. The small clinical and research team comprises a team leader, four sessional psychiatrists, three case managers and two family workers who also undertake community development and group interventions. A range of brochures and a staff procedure manual are available at www.early-psychosis.

Preliminary data on symptom outcome at 1 and 2 years indicate that:

- A significant improvement in positive symptoms occurs by 3 months.
- There is no significant change in negative symptoms over time.
- Depression increases significantly in the first 3 months and then decreases significantly from 3 to 12 months.
- At 1 year, 72% of patients were in remission, 20% continued to be psychotic, and 8% were psychotic but had experienced at least one period of remission.

Prevention through Risk Identification and Management (PRIME)

A research clinic, Prevention through Risk Identification and Management (PRIME), targets individuals considered to be at imminent risk of developing a psychotic disorder. It offers medication trials as well as individual and family therapy.

Education for schools, colleges and family practitioners is provided. The project is part of a study associated with the Yale University.

Based in Connecticut, North Carolina, Toronto and Calgary, PRIME is a randomized double-blind trial for individuals meeting criteria for the prodromal state of psychosis. The study compares olanzapine and placebo in the prevention or postponement of conversions from a prodromal state to an active psychosis. A diagnostic semi-structured interview (the Structured Interview for Prodromal Symptoms – SIPS), and a severity scale (the Scale of Prodromal Symptoms – SOPS) are used to define, diagnose and systematically measure change in individuals who may be prepsychotic (McGlashan et al in press, Miller et al 1999).

The Calgary EPP: a developmental process

"Five years ago the development of our Early Psychosis Program began with the idea that there were many treatments – both pharmacological and psychosocial – that could have a positive impact on schizophrenia. It made sense to consider offering those being diagnosed with the illness all possible treatment options that might be successful. Not only should such a wide range of treatments be offered but these should be offered as soon as possible. *Thus, we began working with the 'first episode'.*

"Referrals came from professionals and from individuals seeking help themselves. They did not all meet criteria for schizophrenia, rather they seemed to have various forms of psychotic illnesses that did not necessarily fit one of the established DSM-IV schizophrenia spectrum diagnoses. *Now we were working with 'early psychosis'.*

"This included treatment options for patients and their families. However, a whole community needed education so that they would understand the notion of psychosis being a range of symptoms for which there were many treatment options and many outcomes – some very favourable. As the community of mental health professionals and lay people become more familiar with psychosis they bring demands for early treatment and possible prevention. *This meant we now addressed early detection and the potential of possible prevention.*

"Our early psychosis programme thus developed from a desire to develop a programme that would offer the best possible treatments at the beginning of the schizophrenia illness to a programme that addresses psychosis in all its forms as early, as thoroughly and as intensely as possible."

Jean Addington

National project site

Calgary is one of three sites for the 'Youth and Mental Illness: Early Intervention' project of the Canadian Mental Health Association, a voluntary organization that aims to improve the quality of life and care for people with mental illnesses. A nurse from EPP and an Association representative are developing a training module for teachers, counsellors and youth workers.

Youth and Mental Illness: Early Intervention project

The Youth and Mental Illness: Early Intervention project is a 26 month national project of the Canadian Mental Health Association, funded by Health Canada, which began in February 1999. The aim is to raise awareness regarding the importance of early intervention in the specific context of youth and psychosis, through:

- development and dissemination of educational resource materials
- facilitation of local early intervention activities at three sites (Calgary, Winnipeg and Fredericton)
- facilitation of a national network of interest and information-sharing

Clinicians from established clinical and research sites in Calgary, Hamilton, London, Toronto and Nova Scotia are among the project advisors. Project materials include pamphlets, an introductory document on early psychosis, project and 'family-to-family' newsletters, a 'parent to parent' support video (*One Day at a Time*), and a booklet describing Canadian early psychosis initiatives. Most of the printed materials are available in English and French at www.cmha.ca. A national policy forum is proposed.

Analysis of service developments

The five models described above have developed in different ways and under different influences. The seeds of EPPIC and TIPS were planted in the 1980s, and these organizations took 6–8 years to evolve into their current forms. The focus of EPPIC is the development of innovative phase-oriented treatment following the onset of psychosis (the 'clinical laboratory' for the study of first-episode psychosis) within a framework of a specialist structure. The basis of TIPS is optimal treatment for schizophrenia within an ordinary treatment organization, with an emphasis on shortening the duration of untreated psychosis through extensive, sustained community education programmes. The Birmingham and Canadian models commenced in the mid-1990s and have much in common with EPPIC (including therapeutic case management and cognitive–behavioural interventions), which to some extent reflects the close communication between members of the programmes.

Each service needs to be considered in the context of the local mental health culture. For example:

- EPPIC operates in the context of Victorian Government Support for 24-hour mobile assessment and treatment teams (www.dhs.vic.gov.au/acmh/mh).

- Norwegian mental health services have a psychodynamic orientation.
- There is a strong emphasis in Canada on consumer and family self-help initiatives.

Over the years, EPPIC and EIS reduced their upper age limit from 45 to 30 years, moving towards a youth model. Both services accept all psychotic disorders, whereas TIPS and the two Canadian programmes have, to date, focused on schizophrenia spectrum disorders, necessitating a broader age range. Themes in the development of these five services include:

- skilled leadership by persistent and committed clinician-researchers who are able to assume multiple roles (Wasylenki and Goering 1995)
- in the early phase of development:
  - needs analyses and pilot studies
  - conferences for mental health workers, administrators, and consumers on 'home turf' with notable visiting speakers as consciousness-raising exercises
  - active dialogue between key players, including site visits
  - written statement of philosophy, principles and vision
  - bids for new or expanded funding
- in the middle phase of development:
  - documentation of service elements
  - assisting and collaborating with other services

- in the later phase of development:
  - examination of outcome data
  - influence on policy

There are now a number of other large-scale early intervention projects in operation around the world, some of which are described in Chapters 6–8.

Thornicroft and Tansella (Tansella and Thornicroft 1998, Thornicroft and Tansella 1999) emphasize the importance of a clear conceptual framework to facilitate the development of mental health. They proposed a matrix model, which defines inputs, processes and outcomes at the level of individual patients, local services, and regions or nations. On reviewing the five models outlined in this chapter, there is a sense that inputs and outcomes have been defined and articulated, but there has been less attention to processes. The initial impetus was to improve outcomes for individual patients, leading to the development of local services. As interest in the specific needs of patients with early psychosis continues to grow, and as research adds depth to clinical experience, local services are beginning to influence regional and national policies. The widespread adoption of early intervention will necessitate monitoring of service provision, using agreed definitions and indicators, and then formal evaluation (see Chapter 7).

Developing an early psychosis service – 'nuts and bolts'

6

There is no absolutely reliable cookbook or bible for developing new systems of care . . . The recipe may vary, and the ingredients may be put together differently in different places, according to demography, culture, government policy and resources. There must always be encouragement to innovate. (Rosen et al 1997, p. 40)

An early psychosis service can be developed in many different ways. Diversity and creativity are to be encouraged, and services should be developed in ways that are congruent and synergistic with the local setting. A vital element in the process is the development of a set of goals. Planning is essential in terms of:

- objectives (what you want to do and why?)
- strategy and tactics (how you will implement the planned changes?)

The paths in developing the early psychosis services outlined in Chapter 5 illustrate the following points:

- Where historical and/or local political factors have been favourable, it has been possible to globally *reform the service system* (e.g. EPPIC and EIS Birmingham) in substantial catchment areas or regions using the argument that there are gaps in existing services.

- Arguments for enhanced services have enabled establishment of *single-component services* such as detection and assessment services, staff training programmes, high-risk clinics, or recent-onset family interventions (e.g. NEPP, Australia).
- *Time-limited research or service projects,* made possible through short-term additional funding, have acted as catalysts to enhance clinical expertise (e.g. the TIPS project). Such projects are either terminated when funding ceases, or are continued from existing resources.
- Features commonly found in *general service systems* can be built upon (e.g. EPPIC Statewide Services *Early Psychosis Projects*). Existing treatment protocols and services can sometimes be refocused or reorganized to cater for the special needs of patients with first-episode psychosis (see Chapter 8).

The nine-step model for developing an early psychosis service, outlined below, is based on an earlier three-step model of 'getting started' (McGorry et al 1999) and the broad seven-step model to reform community services advanced by Thornicroft and Tansella (1999). The steps are not necessarily sequential.

A nine-step model

Step 1: state the philosophy and principles

Philosophy shapes the general organization of a service and *principles* guide specific daily activities. Developing a written statement of philosophy and principles will often involve adaptation and reconfirmation of previously produced declarations. Chapters 1 and 9 should provide guidance, and many of the EPPIC materials referenced in Chapters 2–4 illustrate application of these principles. For broader examples relating to mental health services in general, see Thornicroft and Tansella (1999). Written statements will need to be reviewed periodically, particularly when a service develops significantly or shifts in direction.

> **Sources of information on philosophy and principles of early intervention**
> - Early psychosis books and special editions of journals, including:
>   - Birchwood et al (2000)
>   - McGlashan (1996)
>   - McGorry (1998)
>   - McGorry and Jackson (1999)
> - 'Point of view' academic papers, including:
>   - Birchwood et al (1997)

- Garety and Jolley (2000)
- Klosterkötter (1998)
- Malla and Norman (1999)
- Malla et al (1999)
- Spencer et al (2001) (see commentary by Lewis and Drake 2001)
- Service documents, including:
  - *An Introduction to Early Psychosis Intervention: Some Relevant Findings and Emerging Practices* (www.cmha.ca)
  - *Prevention and Early Intervention Program for Psychosis: Screening, Assessment and Treatment Manuals* (www.pepp.ca)
- 'framework' documents, including:
  - *Early Psychosis Identification and Intervention Initiative: Towards a Framework and Best Practice Approach in Regional Implementation* (www.mheccu.ubc.ca /EPI)
  - *Getting in Early: A Framework for Early Intervention and Prevention in Mental Health for Young People in New South Wales* (New South Wales Health Department 2000b, www.health.nsw.gov.au)
  - *Australian Clinical Guidelines*

for Early Psychosis (National Early Psychosis Project 1998)
- *Early Intervention in Psychosis: Clinical Guidelines and Service Frameworks and Tool Kit* (Initiative to Reduce the Impact of Schizophrenia (IRIS) 2001, www.iris-initiative.org.uk)
- funding applications: services will often provide copies of submissions upon request

Step 2: set the boundary conditions for first-episode psychosis

The incidence of psychotic disorders within the catchment area or sector should be determined. Local epidemiological data are often unavailable and estimates will have to be based on national or international data (see Thornicroft and Tansella 1999). Figures from the World Health Organization (Jablensky et al 1992) provide only a guide because there is a range of incidence rates, particularly for broadly defined schizophrenia (Eaton 1999, Jablensky 1997). Nevertheless, it is useful to obtain estimates of the maximum and minimum levels. Any marked discrepancy between anticipated and actual incidence rates should be noted and considered as a topic for future investigation.

A service will need to determine a policy

on its responsibility for individuals who may be experiencing a prepsychotic prodrome or who are otherwise judged to be at high risk for developing a psychotic illness. If such cases are accepted into a service, then the numbers of cases to be managed is potentially very large.

Age

It is necessary to define an age range on which to focus, which may be:

- adolescents and young adults (for example, 12 or 14 years to 25 or 30 years), based on the concept of youth psychiatry
- linked to the criteria of an associated adult mental health service (for example, 16–45 or 65 years)

About 20% of cases of first-episode psychosis are aged 15–18 years, and onset younger than 14 years is rare.

Age criteria for mental health services are, for the most part, historical, reflecting a traditional division between child and adult psychiatry. Arguments for developing 'youth psychiatry' services need to consider:

- the epidemiology of psychiatric disorders in general and psychotic disorders in particular, for which there is a peak onset in adolescence and early adulthood
- the developmental and subcultural complexity of adolescents.

Partnerships between child and adult psychiatry in the treatment of early psychosis, such as the three examples outlined in the text boxes, deserve serious consideration.

> **Bridging child and adult psychiatry – example 1**
>
> The **Heidelberg Early Adolescent and Adult Recognition and Therapy Center (HEART) for Psychosis**, Germany, was founded in 1996 and involves cooperation between the Departments of Child and Adolescent Psychiatry and Adult Psychiatry. Boundaries of different services often prohibit a common framework of diagnosis and therapy for adolescents (Brunner et al 1998). For example, child psychiatry services provide a range of psychodynamic and/or behavioural psychotherapeutic interventions but frequently lack experience with acute psychotic crises and pharmacological interventions. Adult psychiatry, on the other hand, often lacks skills in the specific psychotherapeutic approach required for this age group.
>
> HEART targets 12–25 year-olds for early recognition and intervention (Resch et al in press). The multi-component service provides

pharmacological interventions, social therapy, family work and individual psychotherapy, with a focus on four elements: symptom reduction, attachment and relationships, developmental tasks, and relapse prevention. A Mobile Support System (MBS) operates as a preventive after care service, engaging patients during the acute phase in preparation for home treatment. The service grew from a pilot project between the acute inpatient unit and child and adult psychiatric services in 1994. Staff and offices are provided by both departments.

Enquiries: franz_resch@med. uni-heidelberg.de or christoph.mundt @med.uni-heidelberg.de

Bridging child and adult psychiatry – example 2
The **Young People, Early Psychosis and Intervention (YPPI) Programme** is a youth-oriented, mobile, community-based service for 14- to 24-year olds experiencing early psychosis living on the central coast of New South Wales, Australia. The

home-based programme includes intensive case management and outreach.

The first phase, initiated in 1994, involved researching the needs of young people with significant mental health problems through a literature review and client survey, followed by identification of best practice models. The second phase commenced with continued funding in July 1995. A subsequent project grant enabled evaluation of the initiative.

Pre- and post-treatment comparisons from 40 YPPI participants indicated a reduction in psychiatric disability, suicidality and depression over 6–12 months. The high level of drug and alcohol use remained unchanged and the team is piloting a specific drug and alcohol intervention. The formal report of the evaluation includes facts sheets, client information pamphlets, sticker, postcard, poster, link-up card and staff training video (Howe et al 1999).

Enquiries: dhowe@doh.health.nsw. gov.au

Bridging child and adult psychiatry – example 3

The **Early Psychosis Intervention (EPI) Program**, in the South Fraser region of British Columbia, Canada, aims to bridge the youth/adult division for individuals aged 13–30 years who have first-episode psychosis or an 'at-risk mental state' through an inter-ministerial 'portfolio holders' model. In British Columbia, child and youth mental health services are managed by a provincial government ministry, but adult mental health services are managed by regional health boards. Community mental health teams in both youth services and adult services have designated psychiatrists and mental health clinicians who provide treatment and case management for early psychosis.

The EPI Program has a single intake clinician, and a psychiatrist is available for urgent psychiatric assessments and follow up. Youth and adults diagnosed with first-episode psychosis are then treated by the appropriate portfolio holders, according to locality and age. Psychoeducation groups are available for adolescents, young adults and family members.

Enquiries: karen.tee@gems4.gov. bc.ca or bill.macewan@ southfraserhealth.com

Disorders

Definition of the boundaries of first-episode psychosis must include the diagnostic groups to be targeted. This might include only non-affective psychoses (e.g. TIPS, PEPP, and EPP Calgary, described in Chapter 5) or all psychotic disorders (e.g. EPPIC and EPS Birmingham, described in Chapter 5). In first-episode psychosis the diagnosis is often unclear in the early stages (Fennig et al 1994, Strakowski 1994), but premature exclusion of patients initially thought to have psychosis associated with mood or personality disorders might lead to a longer duration of untreated psychosis in those who are mis-classified.

EPPIC example

- The estimated resident population of EPPIC's catchment area was 852 000 in June 1999 (Australian Bureau of Statistics 2000), with 206 279 aged 15–29 years. The number of people aged 15–29 was estimated to increase by 0.8% annually over the next decade

(Victorian Department of Infrastructure 2000).

- A mid-range figure of 10 per 10 000 was used for the total estimated incidence of new cases of affective *and* nonaffective psychoses in the EPPIC catchment area, based on WHO incidence rates for schizophrenia spectrum diagnoses in 15–24 year olds, amounting to about 200 cases per year (Edwards and McGorry 1998). The EPPIC intake data for 1995–1996 indicated a rate of 11.44 cases per 10 000 people per year in the 15–29 year age group (Power et al 1998).

- Based on the 1995–1996 figures approximately 236 new cases would be expected each year (i.e. 206 279 × 11.4/10 000). In fact, between 1997 and 2000 the number of new cases of first-episode psychosis accepted by EPPIC averaged 255 cases per year (Amminger et al, 2002).

Step 3: assess the population needs and current service use

Once the estimated numbers of cases of first-episode psychosis have been obtained, the specific needs of this group in the local setting need to be clarified both quantitatively and qualitatively. For example:

- How many early psychosis cases do the mental health services currently have registered?
- Based on incidence estimates, how many cases are probably not being treated by mental health services?
- Are these 'missing' patients being serviced by private mental health services or by primary care physicians, or not being treated at all? Are there opportunities for collaboration with these other service providers?
- What were the existing patients' pathways to care, the duration of untreated psychosis, and patients' and families' experience of treatment?
- How long do patients stay in treatment?
- Is there continuity of care? How many different case managers or doctors does a young persons see over a 12-month period?
- Is there a need for written materials in multiple languages?

Qualitative study beginnings

In a quest to improve early intervention across the province of British Columbia, Canada, the Ministry for Health and Ministry for

Children and Families combined with consumer and family advocacy organizations and major service provider organizations to launch the **Early Psychosis Initiative (EPI)** (www.mheccu.uba.ca). The Initiative was informed by the British Columbia Early Intervention Study (www.cmha-bc.org), a qualitative study of people's first experiences with mental illness and the mental health system.

EPI commenced in 1999 funded by a grant from the Ministry of Health, and funding was provided by both Ministries in subsequent years. The Mental Health Evaluation and Community Consultation Unit (M*heccu*) was contracted to implement EPI with guidance from an inter-ministry working group.

The primary goal of EPI was to establish regional initiatives to improve identification and intervention for young person with early signs and symptoms of psychosis. The initiatives included five demonstration projects, ranging from evaluation of existing rural programmes to implementation of early psychosis programmes. Strategically targeted education initiatives included:

- establishment of EPI committees in all 18 health regions within the province, to examine service delivery and referral pathways, and to educate management about early intervention
- early identification education aimed at 'gatekeepers' such as general practitioners
- clinical skill-building aimed at physicians and mental health professionals

Training materials include pamphlets, booklets for physicians and mental health clinicians, *Reaching Out* videos for physicians, school and community use, a train-the-trainer manual and a television commercial. A teacher's manual aimed at high school students was developed by the British Columbia Schizophrenia Society, containing an outline and support materials for a one- or two-period lesson (bcss@istar.ca). Consumers, represented on most of the 18 regional committees, are involved in reviewing all materials and educational events. *A Practical Guide to Care in Early Psychosis*, a service evaluation report and a policy document are in preparation.

Auditing services at baseline – example 1

Tobin and Chen (1999) describe a quality improvement process involving an audit of 14 cases of early psychosis presenting to a mental health service in an outer suburban area of Sydney, Australia. In addition, a consumer survey was designed to assess whether nine best-practice interventions had occurred and whether they subjectively were considered useful to the consumer or carer. This audit was undertaken in preparation for the formation of early psychosis treatment guidelines for the service (see Chapter 7).

Auditing services at baseline – example 2

The Worcestershire Community and Mental Health NHS Trust in the UK audited clinical management of first-episode psychosis cases over the previous 3 years. Information was collected on pathways to care, duration of untreated psychosis, prescribing practices, care plans, engagement, and professional and other contacts. The data will be compared with best-practice

guidelines for early intervention to identify strengths and target potential areas for change when developing local early intervention services.

Primary care physicians are the 'gatekeepers' to care in most health systems, and are often the first professionals contacted for help by patients concerned about their mental health. Their role is essential in the early recognition and initial treatment of psychosis (Lincoln and McGorry 1999, Macmillan and Shiers 2000). One of the first tasks in establishing an early psychosis service is to evaluate the links between existing mental health service and primary care physicians and, if necessary, improve them. Specialist services need to embrace the challenge of educating primary care networks, in a structured and methodical way, about the early detection of psychosis and appropriate intervention. Such education should, ideally, be part of a broader strategy to strengthen primary mental health care and/or youth mental health.

Step 4: set the early psychosis scene

Staff training

A key tactic in developing an early psychosis service is to provide training in it for staff in existing mental health services. If this occurs early in the process it can act as a catalyst for stimulating interest in the service and also provide valuable feedback on attitudes to, and expertise in, early psychosis.

Bureaucrats and politicians

The level of support and capacity of health planners, administrators and politicians to respond to the challenge is a key variable in establishing an early psychosis service, since it determines the resources that will be available through new funding or reallocation of existing resources. Consultation with health planners, policy makers and management groups helps to sell the concept. This process is often the rate-limiting step for substantial and durable change in services. Politicians respond to community pressure, and the influence of the electoral cycle should be kept in mind. Leaders in the early psychosis field can be requested to spend time with senior bureaucrats and politicians to support the case for specialist services, and to sow the seeds for the medium- to long-term objective of policy development.

Academics

Some early psychosis programmes have developed within the context of a university setting (e.g. the Adolescent Clinic at the Amsterdam Medical Clinic, Developmental Processes in the Early Course of Illness in Los Angeles, the Program for Assessment and Care of Early Schizophrenia in Pittsburgh – see Edwards et al 2000 for descriptions of these three services). Others have been developed by staff in standard public mental health services, sometimes in discussion with academic departments with a view to collaborative research.

Relating research to clinical practice is a major challenge (Dawson 1997). Projects that are research driven can be limited in their clinical impact, whereas innovative service delivery initiatives lacking research components are often difficult to sustain. The preparedness of researchers to assume multiple roles in service delivery (Wasylenki and Goering 1995) can help to reduce the gap between science and practice.

Raising awareness

The attitude and morale of local clinicians and their potential to respond positively to innovation is an important element in establishing a first-episode psychosis service. If there is a positive attitude and high morale, then it is likely their enthusiasm can be mobilized readily if resources are obtained to initiate reform, and it may prove to be a powerful force for change. The level of interest of local clinicians can be assessed through the response to awareness-raising lectures and workshops on early psychosis. The early intervention strategy involves rekindling and harnessing the altruism and energies of mental health workers, which may have become blunted.

Communication with other services

Visits to other early psychosis services, establishing links with staff in those services and accessing their resource materials can be valuable. A 'serial leverage' process often occurs, in which staff in a service use the experience of others to develop their own ideas, leading to a positive feedback cycle at both clinical and organizational level. An example is the ongoing dialogue between TIPS (see Chapter 5) and EPPIC over a period of at least 6 years, regarding community education about psychosis (see the Compass Project, Chapter 2).

There are sizeable projects in the four cities (Auckland, Wellington, Christchurch and Dunedin) and some services are delivered within a Maori (indigenous New Zealander) cultural framework. Annual training forums are organized and a national research and evaluation protocol is being considered. The provision of early intervention services is recommended in the *Blueprint for Mental Health Services in New Zealand* (Mental Health Commission 1998).

Enquiries: davidb@healthotago.co.nz

Communication between projects – example 1

The **New Zealand National Early Intervention Interest Group** developed a document to guide service funders about the clinical and organizational steps needed to provide specialist early psychosis programmes. The success of lobbying for funding during a 5-year period is reflected in a directory of 19 early psychosis services currently operating in New Zealand.

Communication between projects – example 2

The **Swiss Early Psychosis Project (SWEPP)** is a forum to encourage national collaboration in developing intervention and research strategies for early psychosis. Educational activities are organized, including an education programme for general practitioners, and information about new developments is provided through a website (www.come.to/swepp).

Communication between projects – example 3
The **European First Episode Schizophrenia Network (Euro FESN)** is an informal network of interested scientists in Europe. Aggregation of data from patients with a first episode of psychosis provides an epidemiological basis for phenomenological, cognitive and biological investigations, access to treatment-naive patients, representative outcome studies, and a focus for early intervention studies. The aims are:

- to raise the international profile of schizophrenia research
- to exchange information about sampling strategies, assessment instruments, imaging and image analysis protocols, and intervention methods
- to promote national and international collaborations in first-episode research, particularly for large samples, rare subgroups, and cross-national comparisons of intervention and outcome

A list of network members and meeting reports are available at www.man.ac.uk/~mdphwnj/fesn1.html. A consensus on best practice in first-episode psychosis was developed by Euro FESN at a meeting in Davos, Switzerland, in February 2000, and is contained in Appendix 3.

Enquiries: shon.lewis@man.ac.uk

International Early Psychosis Association (IEPA)
The IEPA was conceived at the First International Conference for Preventive Strategies in Early Psychosis held in Melbourne, Australia, in 1996, recognizing the need for an international organization to facilitate collaborative initiatives and promote best practice in the field of early psychosis. The IEPA web site includes information on early psychosis initiatives, conferences, and chat groups (www.iepa.org.au). By March 2001 the IEPA had 1647 members from 57 countries.

Enquiries: iepa@vicnet.net.au

Community psychiatric nurses report on a site visit
"We had the opportunity to visit EPPIC after receiving a bursary award

through our Northamptonshire NHS Trust (United Kingdom). From our first day of our two-week visit we were acutely aware of the overwhelming sense of optimism that ran through all aspects of the service delivery. A variety of teams were working together like 'cogs in a clock' to provide a comprehensive and cohesive service. There was a positive atmosphere of 'can do' when faced with difficult situations. Services were developed to meet the needs of individuals rather than fitting individuals into available services.

"To maximise the experience of visiting an early intervention service we recommend prior knowledge of the early psychosis literature and some experience in clinical application. Visiting EPPIC 'in vivo' enabled us to reflect on our own service and consider consolidation. The knowledge that we have gained through this has given us the credibility within our NHS Trust to drive service development.

"In addition to our longer-term objective of setting up an early intervention service at home, it seemed imperative to quickly provide a concrete example of applying the principles we had learnt. To this end,

within a month of our return from Australia, we started the process of providing a 'family and friends' psychoeducation group. We hope that by demonstrating that this work isn't 'rocket science' our colleagues will be instilled with the enthusiasm and confidence that the visit engendered in us and will work alongside us to develop our service in the future."

Early psychosis resources

Gather written and visual resource materials and disseminate these to clinicians, researchers, and managers. Academic papers, practical manuals or patient information tools such as videos and web site addresses can be highly influential. At a later stage, a strategy is needed to make these resources readily available for clinicians to use with patients and their families.

Step 5: identify an early psychosis workforce

Clinicians capable of driving or facilitating an early psychosis service need to be identified. Potential participants may declare themselves during staff training activities. People with particular skills (e.g. organizational, psychosocial, research) may need encouragement to become involved, as it is important to have a range of disciplines represented in the endeavour. Harnessing the interest of nursing leaders is critical in terms of developing the early psychosis philosophy and influencing inpatient care.

Resources needed to support the project, especially in terms of clinical supervision and training, must be defined. Do interested individuals have relevant expertise? Could some people develop the required expertise relatively easily through reading and site visits? Examine the potential for collaborative ventures with neighbouring services in training and supervision.

Additional resources

Attracting additional funding to catalyse a restructure of the service and enhance clinical expertise can be a powerful influence. It is often difficult to pursue a new initiative without some allocation of dedicated resources. However, it is sometimes easier to secure grants when a project has commenced and pilot data on outcomes are available. Securing sessional clinical input for a limited time – a relatively inexpensive manoeuvre – can be helpful in the early stages. Academics who have an interest in early psychosis can be encouraged to undertake sabbaticals in affiliation with early psychosis initiatives.

Step 6: define the focus

Options

It is important to be clear about the potential focus of the proposed service. At the most basic level there is a distinction to be made between services oriented to the prepsychotic/prodrome phase and those oriented to first-episode psychosis. The objectives, strategies, ethical issues and professional responsibilities in these domains vary significantly. Shortening the duration of untreated psychosis is another possible focus. However, the need to improve the quality of treatment in first-episode psychosis and during the early critical years of illness is perhaps the strongest reason for reorganizing services. This may involve the provision of comprehensive expert treatment, reduction in the duration of active psychosis in the first episode and beyond, and attempts to maximize recovery, reintegration and quality of life.

Figure 6.1 provides examples of early intervention strategies structured by phase of illness (prodromal or active psychosis) and the patient's position in the care pathway. Interventions that focus on the prodrome and duration of untreated psychosis tend to be research driven (see Larsen et al 2001a, for a review of published studies). There are many projects on the prodromal stage under development, and results of recent initiatives will start to be reported in the next few years.

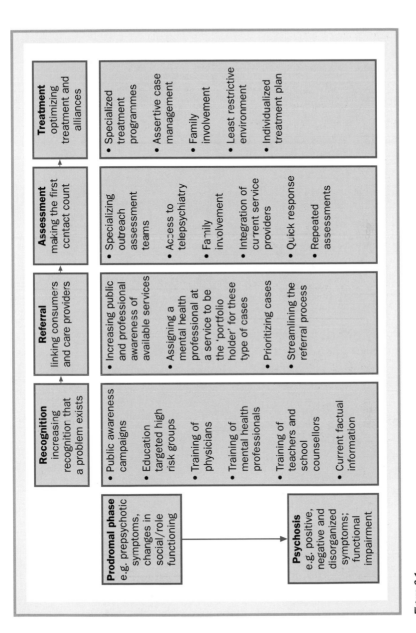

Figure 6.1
Optimal strategies in pathways to care.
Adapted with permission of Mental Health Evaluation and Community Consultation Unit (Mheccu), from Mheccu (1999) Early Psychosis Identification and Intervention Initiative: Towards a Framework and Best Practice Approach in Regional Implementation.

Focus on prodrome, Germany

The **Early Recognition and Intervention for Psychotic Disorders** project in Cologne aims to recognize people at high risk of developing psychosis and to intervene to prevent progression (FETZ; www.fetz.org). Individuals are included on the basis of symptoms, family history and neurobiological abnormalities. Participants are randomly assigned to treatment (a combination of pharmacological and psychosocial therapy) or a control group. The target group is aged 18 years or more and 120 new cases will be accepted each year. The estimated total case load is 150 individuals receiving 2-monthly follow up.

The FETZ project is a recruiting centre for Network of Competence (Kompetenz-Netz) for Schizophrenia, a 5-year research programme funded by the German government. Projects related to prodrome include:

- development of the Early Recognition Inventory (ERI) which is based on the IRAOS (see Chapter 3)
- biological markers of psychosis
- psychological interventions in the early prodrome
- pharmacological interventions in the late prodrome
- biological foundations of early pharmacological interventions
- an awareness programme.

Other recruiting centres are located in Bonn, Munich and Dusseldorf.

Enquiries: beratung@fetz.org or projekleitung@fetz.org

Focus on duration of untreated psychosis and treatment, Denmark

A project on the early identification and treatment of young psychotic patients, **OPUS**, is in progress in Copenhagen and Århus, Denmark. It is examining whether the duration of untreated psychosis can be shortened and whether early detection leads to better outcomes (Jørgensen et al 2000). Each city is divided into areas in which detection will be improved or usual practice will continue. Additionally, patients are randomized to usual treatment or integrated care with a psychosis team for a 2-year period. Integrated care comprises assertive community treatment, psychoeducational multi-family groups, and social skills training. A third option is provided for inpatients in Copenhagen – admission to a special first-episode psychosis unit, U7.

In a 3-year inclusion period (1998–2000), 578 people aged 18–45 years with non-affective first-episode were included. Comprehensive follow-up interviews were conducted at 1-year and 2-years. Analysis of 1-year follow-up data obtained from the first 341 participants showed that reduction in psychotic symptoms was greater for patients in the integrated care group, and that patients and families in this group were more involved and more satisfied with treatment (Nordentoft et al, in press). A five-year follow-up is planned.

Enquiries: OPUS – merete.nordentoft @dadlnet.dk; U7 – soeren.bredkjaer@ shh.hosp.dk

Focus on prodrome and treatment, Australia

The **Psychological Assistance Service** (**PAS**) in the Hunter Valley of New South Wales identifies young people at risk of developing a psychotic disorder, provides assessment and treatment to those at high risk of psychosis or experiencing a first episode of psychosis, and provides consultation to relevant services (Carr et al 2000). The region includes about 120 000 people in the target age group of 14–30 years. The service developed from a pilot staff education programme in first-episode psychosis.

Follow-up evaluations were undertaken for 23 'at-risk' patients at an average of 14.6 months after initial assessment. Only 9% developed a psychotic episode. The relatively low transition rate may reflect the inclusion of second-degree relatives in the 'trait' at-risk group and, in some cases, insufficient follow-up periods (range 4–34 months).

Enquiries: hunterpas@doh.health. nsw.gov.au

Scoping

Data from a needs assessment can assist in defining the focus of a proposed early psychosis service. For example, are the numbers of first-episode psychosis high enough to warrant the development of a dedicated service? If not, a joint venture with neighbouring services may be an option. Is there a relatively high number of young people with established or chronic psychotic illness? If so, a greater emphasis on prevention and early intervention may be appropriate.

Mental health service catchment areas typically include 40 000 to 150 000 people. Existing first-episode psychosis services commonly cover a region or city including 300 000 to 1 million residents. If a smaller catchment area is used, then viable numbers of patients might be maintained by extending the follow-up period.

In rural or remote areas it may be necessary to target young people with psychotic disorders, including those who have experienced multiple episodes, rather than focusing exclusively on first-episode cases. This might achieve a critical mass of recent-onset cases. Models adopted by the Scandinavian countries (Alanen et al 1994) and the initiatives spawned by the NEPP (see Chapter 5) provide examples of how a critical mass can be achieved.

The time that patients remain within an early psychosis service before transfer to another agency needs to be considered. This period will depend on the level of specialization and whether the service is segregated from mainstream mental health services. A focus on early psychosis, by definition, requires that services are targeted at the 'critical period' following the onset of illness (Birchwood and Macmillan 1993). For example, treatment at EPPIC is provided for 18 months only, leading to a total case load of 400 patients. This time frame is limited by resources and is not ideal (3–5 years would be an improvement), but it allows for the detection, acceptance and management of all new cases within the catchment area. Changes in the size of the catchment area, the age criteria or staff levels would mean that the time frame would have to be reassessed.

Resources

It is possible to create an early psychosis focus or service even if resources are limited. Possible levels of development are depicted in Figure 6.2. Within the area of enhanced targeted models, activities could include a detection and assessment service, improving community awareness about psychosis, a strategy targeting young people with slow or prolonged recovery, a staff development and training programme, or family intervention for recent-onset cases.

Where financial resources are provided for only a limited time, it may be preferable to avoid establishing structures that the general mental health service will not be able to support in the future. Focusing on training may be best in these circumstances, unless funding for continuation of new service can be attracted or the service can be reconfigured to move resources from elsewhere. Another option is to focus on policies and procedures, developing treatment protocols that can be incorporated into mainstream systems.

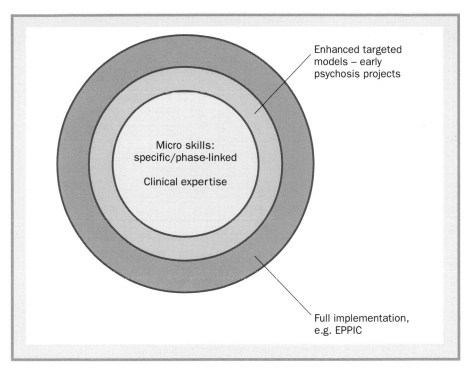

Figure 6.2
Spheres of action for preventive intervention in early psychosis.
Adapted with permission of Gardiner-Caldwell Communications Ltd, from McGorry, PD, Edwards J (1997) Early
Psychosis Training Pack. *Macclesfield, Cheshire: Gardiner-Caldwell.*

Step 7: develop a written plan

A plan outlining short- and long-term objectives, the consultation process, costings, and a timetable should be formulated. Ideally, a pilot phase of operation with evaluation of outcome should be included.

The development process
The preparation work for the **Hong Kong Early Assessment Service for Young People with Psychosis (EASY)** was active and intense, occurring over 6 months (www.ha.org.hk/easy). Four teams of five staff (a psychiatrist,

a medical officer and three psychiatric nurses) plus a psychologist and researcher have been funded to cover Hong Kong (population 7 million). The target group is people aged 15–25 years with any psychotic conditions, and the focus is detection and education. There is no separate inpatient facility. The following time line gives an idea of the numerous steps towards, and influences on, a project that commenced in mid-2001.

1997

- Commencement of a 3-year project measuring duration of untreated psychosis.

1998

- Workshop by EPPIC to introduce concepts and practice to mental health professionals.
- Paper on the rationale for early intervention published in the *Hong Kong Medical Journal* (Chen 1998).

1999

- Interim finding of long duration of untreated psychosis (mean 480 days, median 120 days, 50% longer than 6 months, 33% longer than 1 year) (Chen et al 1999).
- Initial discussion with a non-governmental organization for a pilot project (did not proceed).

2000

- Local symposium with early intervention team from Shanghai, China.
- Working group established in Hong Kong Schizophrenia Research Society for informal discussion.
- Application for research development funding declined.
- Decision to launch pilot projects without extra resources, which involved negotiation and winning the support of colleagues in existing units and identification of key personnel.
- Sponsorship obtained for four members of the Schizophrenia Research Society to attend the International Early Psychosis Association conference in New York.
- Planning and establishment of pilots – naming of programme, development of screening procedure and treatment guidelines, negotiation of interface with child psychiatry team, preparation of educational material and web site, initiation of projects at Queen Mary Hospital and Kwai Chung Hospital.

- Media reported findings on duration of untreated psychosis.
- Government invited submission for new initiative – proposal advanced after informal communication with policy makers, gaining initial approval and negotiating staff resources.
- Presentation of evidence-based material to Hong Kong Hospital Authority Head Office.
- Presentation to Hong Kong Academy of Medicine.
- Formation of working group under a clinical coordinating committee for psychiatry.

2001
- Endorsement of working group report.
- Steering committee established to set strategic outlines.
- Working group established to prepare protocol, education material, etc.
- Four local committees established to advise on implementation and logistics for each team.
- Four team members spend a month at EPPIC for training.

Enquiries: Eric Chen – eyhchen@hku.hk

Step 8: implement key service components

Go for it!

Step 9: monitor and review

Systems for monitoring and review should be in place from the earliest stages of implementing an early psychosis project. The documents produced by the Rockingham/Kwinana Early Psychosis Project are illustrative (see text box).

Monitor and review

The **Rockingham/Kwinana Early Psychosis Project** in Western Australia targets first-episode psychosis patients aged 18–40 years in a catchment area of 90 000. The project, involving 4.5 full-time staff, manages 50–60 patients and their families for a 2-year period. A partnership between the local Division of General Practice, a non-governmental agency, child and adolescent, and adult mental health services has been developed over a 6-year period.

1994
- Health authority formed a reference group to advise on developing services for young people with first-episode psychosis.

1995
- Document completed which outlined a new service model – a culmination of 9 months of planning.
- Funding approved for a 2-year pilot project.
- Steering committee established to oversee the project.
- Functional brief prepared.

1996
- Pilot service commenced.

1997
- Document completed describing operational guidelines and policies.
- Evaluation and review of early psychosis programmes commissioned by the Mental Health Division of the Health Department of Western Australia.
- Report into the 12-month efficacy of the Early Psychosis Project completed by organizational psychologist.

1998
- Recurrent funding secured.
- Guidelines for clinical practice outlined how the system of care operates.

1999
- Early psychosis case management manual produced.

As noted by Catts et al (in press),

The first two years will be occupied by learning 'how to do it', training staff, making service adjustments, and developing a highly structured intervention and evaluation protocol . . . The following two years will be needed to run the protocol without varying it, so that evaluation can occur.

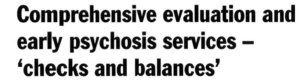

Comprehensive evaluation and early psychosis services – 'checks and balances'

7

It is a considerable burden to develop a service and evaluate it at the same time . . . The next step may now be to manualise the specific aspects of the intervention and to carefully evaluate them, possibly using randomised controlled trials. (Howe et al 1999, p. 202)

Findings on the impact of early intervention must be replicated, while controlling for treatment content. A study of this nature would probably require a quasi-experimental research design. Ethical and other practical considerations would probably preclude a randomized controlled design. Given the widespread variation in systems for delivering mental health services across regions, a parallel control design in two jurisdictions would likely introduce more systematic confounders than would be encountered in a historical control design. (Malla et al 1999, p. 845).

Description and documentation of the theoretical and evidence bases for a particular programme, the goals and aims, and the details of service delivery in each treatment area is critical. This ensures not only that programme staff are aware of their responsibilities in designing and delivering care plans, but also allows external agencies to critically appraise and replicate a programme. Evaluation, encompassing both 'quality control' and outcome assessment, is of key importance, not only for its intrinsic value, but also:

- to satisfy management and funding bodies (Andrews et al 1995)
- as a tool to influence other clinicians and policy makers
- to ensure finite resources are deployed efficiently and for the purposes for which they were intended

Early psychosis projects that integrate programme description and evaluation into everyday service delivery are in an excellent position to demonstrate the integrity of treatments provided, the impact on clients' mental health, and the professionalism and value of their service. This chapter expands on the five-phase approach to programme description and evaluation, based on Owen and Rogers (1999), which has been adopted by EPPIC: description, clarification, programme monitoring, process evaluation, and outcome evaluation (see Figure 7.1). The focus is on treatment integrity, often neglected in the hot pursuit for outcome data.

Describing the service model

Descriptions of the service can be developed over time, with progressive refinement of draft documents. A broad description of the service is a good starting point, and preparing a descriptive paper for publication can add an element of rigour to the task. Alternatively, there may be opportunities to publish in journals that are receptive to discussion of service delivery issues without necessarily presenting data. More detailed descriptions of the service will be required later in the development of the programme, in order to ensure the integrity of treatment. Documents prepared by existing services can be used as a guide.

Journals that may be receptive to descriptive papers include:

- *Advances in Psychiatric Treatment* (http://apt.rcpsych.org)
- *Australasian Psychiatry* (www.blackwell-science.com)
- *Australian and New Zealand Journal of Psychiatry* (www.blackwell-science.com)
- *Journal of Mental Health* (www.carfax.co.uk/jmh-ad.htm)
- *Journal of Psychiatric and Mental Health Nursing* (www.blackwell-science.com)
- *Journal of Psychosocial Nursing* (www.slackinc.com)

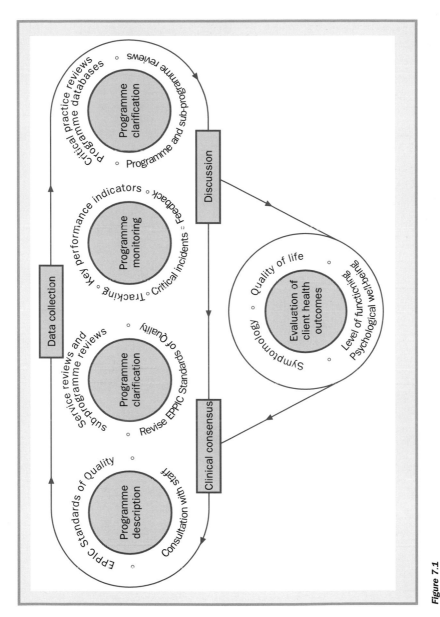

Figure 7.1
A comprehensive framework for evaluation in an early psychosis service.

- *Journal of Psychiatric Rehabilitation* (www.bu.edu/prj)
- *Journal of Psychiatric Rehabilitation Skills* (www.ucpsychrehab.org/publications/journal)
- *Psychiatric Bulletin* (http://pb/rcpsych.org)
- *Psychiatric Services* (http://psychservices.psychiatryonline.org)

Descriptive accounts of other services can assist in providing a framework for written reports. The published accounts of the services outlined in the text boxes provide examples.

Published service descriptions – example 1

The **Psychotic Disorders Team (PDT)** operating in Hamilton, Ontario, Canada, offers intense clinical involvement to individuals with first-episode psychosis and aged 16–65 years in a catchment area of 120 000. The service focuses on:

- early intervention
- helping people to maintain social roles
- reducing trauma and stigma
- psychoeducation
- low-dose antipsychotic therapy

The team of five staff create a

'therapeutic partnership' between the patient, family and clinical team (Hamilton Wilson and Hobbs 1995, Hobbs et al 1999), focusing on short-term goals. A family educator provides support, education and advocacy for family members (Hamilton Wilson and Hobbs 1999). Discharged clients are referred to as 'alumni' and ongoing shared care is provided by PDT with the family physician. A study is under way to compare the outcomes of 30 patients who received services from the PDT for a period of 18 months and 30 controls treated by the community's usual network of psychiatric care providers.

Published service descriptions – example 2

The **Early Psychosis Programme**, Nova Scotia, Canada, established in 1995 as a partnership between the Nova Scotia Hospital and the Dalhousie University Department of Psychiatry, provides assessment and outpatient treatment for new patients aged 15–20 years with non-affective psychosis, in a catchment area of 900 000 (www.nshospital.ns.ca/rehabilitation.html#programs). Key treatment components include (Whitehorn et al 1998):

- an attitude of hope, optimism and respect
- early treatment with second-generation antipsychotic agents
- psychoeducation and counselling
- help in returning to vocational and educational activities
- active involvement of families

Educational activities for mental health professionals occur through the Early Psychosis Mentorship Program of bimonthly workshops, site visits, and an annual conference. An 8-week multi-family group and ongoing family support group operate, and a sibling support group is planned. A video *The Sooner the Better* (margie.crown@nshospital. ns.ca) assists the education process. Research focuses on brain structure and function, trials of new antipsychotic agents, and descriptions of patterns of recovery. In the process of reorganizing the local health care system, the service has been identified as a model programme and is likely to receive improved funding, in part due to lobbying by family members.

Published service descriptions – example 3

The **Southern Area First Episode (SAFE) Project**, New South Wales, Australia, was initiated to develop best practice protocols suited to the needs and resources of a small rural mental health service (population of 182 000 across 52 000 square kilometres) in New South Wales, Australia (Welch and Garland 2000, ausinet.flinders. edu.au/stocktake2/stoc0097.htm). It involved the following steps:

- Two clinicians from each of the child and adolescent and adult mental health teams were trained and supervised by established services to become experts in the identification, assessment and treatment of first-episode psychosis.
- These four clinicians gradually assumed case loads, with supervision occurring through teleconferencing and site visits.
- In collaboration with the project team, guidelines were developed which formed the basis of an education and training package designed to enhance basic skills of clinicians working in the area.

- A 'mainstreaming process' commenced in which groups (e.g. mental health workers, general practitioners, school counsellors) were targeted for education and training, including a strategic series of 1- and 2-day workshops.

Additional staff have now undergone similar training to ensure broad coverage of the region. The role of specialist clinicians will change over time, with encouragement of all staff to undertake early psychosis work with support and clinical supervision.

Describing the treatments that a new programme intends to offer clients, or documenting the treatment approach that has evolved, is time consuming and challenging.

Suggested documentation for an early psychosis programme
- pathways to care
- prodromal interventions
- principles of treatment:
  - least restrictive interventions (e.g. criteria for inpatient care versus home treatment)
  - joint care planning
  - responsibilities of clinical staff
- inpatient and outpatient treatment

in the acute and recovery phases:
  - how often are clients seen?
  - what are the goals of the care plan?
  - what is the focus of sessions?
  - medication strategies and other medical interventions
- crisis support
- psychological interventions
- psychoeducation
  - how and when are concepts introduced?
  - what supporting material is provided?
- family work
- other psychosocial interventions (e.g. groups, vocational sessions)

Clinicians will vary – either appropriately or inappropriately – in the way they deliver services to individuals (Grimshaw and Hutchinson 1995). The EPPIC Standards of Quality were developed to formalize the components of clinical care considered relevant to best practice in early psychosis (see EPPIC 2001b). Developed in consultation with EPPIC staff, with consideration of the programme's guiding philosophies, and grouped according to illness phase, the Standards aim to create practice guidelines that identify minimum essential components of clinical practice. Quantifiable indicators have been derived (see Table 7.1).

Table 7.1
Sample from EPPIC Standards of Quality (EPPIC 2001b)

Standard	Indicator
The OCM* should have at least fortnightly contact with patients; rationale for variations in the frequency of appointments should be clearly indicated in the notes	• Average number of OCM contacts per patient
History and case formulation, including provisional diagnosis and management plan, should be completed within 6 weeks	• Of files with case formulation, provisional diagnosis and management plan present
Patients with enduring positive symptoms 3 months after entry will be referred to TREAT†	• Number of patients referred to TREAT per month • Percentage of clients who have been in service for at least 3 months who have been referred to TREAT
Referring agents will be contacted by written correspondence and informed of management plan within 6 weeks by the OCM	• Percentage of cases in which this notification exists in the file
Families of patients should be seen at least monthly during early recovery	• Mean number of times family is seen

*OCM, Outpatient case manager.
†TREAT, Treatment Resistant Early Assessment Team.

A framework for programme evaluation

Evaluation is concerned with understanding *how* a programme works, and *how well* it works. The objectives, design and methodology of evaluation in an early psychosis service will differ depending on issues such as:

• how the service model has been developed

• the focus of the evaluation, such as programme implementation or client outcomes
• the broader rationale for the evaluation, for example programme improvement, accountability or research on treatment effectiveness

Clarificative evaluation

Clarificative evaluation aims to clarify

fundamental questions about what the programme or subprogramme is designed to do, and how the service should strive towards meeting its goals. Over time, EPPIC has developed and expanded and experienced pressures common to mental health services such as staff turnover, blurring of subprogramme roles, and internally and externally driven organizational change. These factors can result in changes to the model and distort understanding of the rationale underlying a programme. Service-wide reviews, involving all levels of clinical and support staff, are used to ensure that:

- the approaches to clinical practice are consistent with the philosophical underpinnings
- the service model is implemented appropriately and comprehensively
- staff are clear about the rationale on which the service model is based.

Annual review days are held off-site, chaired by an external facilitator, to discuss the integrity, strengths and weaknesses of the existing service model, and organizational structure. Individual subprogrammes also regularly conduct half- or full-day reviews, often twice yearly, to critically review policy and procedures and discuss matters that are team specific (see text box). Agendas are constructed by team coordinators in collaboration with the facilitator, and approval

is then sought from the programme executive to proceed.

Examples of EPPIC review day agendas

Youth Access Team review topics included:

- the youth model of mental health services
- review of criteria for admission to EPPIC services
- progress in meeting service indicators
- report from an International Early Psychosis Conference
- implementation of a new 'hub and spoke' model for delivering services

Outpatient Case Management review topics included:

- EPPIC model – history and rationale
- plan for working with general practitioners
- development of a case management handbook

Another technique used to clarify aims, standards and interventions is the annual review of the EPPIC Standards within staff development sessions. Clinical staff attend and contribute their own views regarding the appropriateness (or otherwise) of particular standards in light of factors that influence service delivery.

Programme monitoring

Programme monitoring involves the systematic collation of information to evaluate how a programme is being delivered, often with reference to established targets and standards. For example, data are extracted from a number of sources regularly to monitor the performance of EPPIC and its subprogrammes. A number of clinical information systems contain key patient information (e.g. demographics and registration dates) and have been configured to output data regarding referral rates, client characteristics, registrations, discharges and

case loads of staff (see the example in Table 7.2). Data are also accessed from a Victorian state-wide mental health database into which EPPIC staff, like all Victorian public mental health services, input information on clinical activity. Key performance indicator data, including critical incidents, seclusions, contacts, admissions, bed occupancy and 28-day readmission rates, are scrutinized as part of a regional mental health service quality assurance process. This process provides useful experience in collating, understanding and interpreting routine statistics, and examining reasons for deviation from standards and variations over time. Ideally, comparison of key performance indicators against thresholds or benchmarks would also occur within a network of first-episode psychosis services.

Regular quality assurance meetings at EPPIC provide a forum to review programme and subprogramme data, and to undertake an

Table 7.2
Extract from EPPIC caseload report

	Maximum case load	Current case load	Discharges due in 3 months	Discharges overdue	No. of referrals in past 3 months
Team A					
Case Manager P	25	19	1	0	7
Case Manager Q	30	33	6	3	5
Team B					
Case Manager X	10	9	1	2	3
Case Manager Y	15	17	2	1	2

in-depth examination of individual subprogrammes on a rotating schedule. Discussions focus on issues such as intake criteria and guidelines for working with programme components or external services.

Other data are used on a day-to-day basis for programme management purposes. For example, a case-load management report generated by the clinical information system provides subprogramme coordinators with information about current case loads and pending discharges for all case management staff. This facilitates the allocation of case managers and doctors to new EPPIC clients.

or subprogramme coordinators) and a member of the clinical programme being reviewed. Using a pro forma approach, illustrated by the questions in the text box, the reviewers identify common or systemic problems in service delivery. Strategies to improve practice are implemented through the quality assurance structure, nested within the clinical management team. Practice reviews have led to improvements in ongoing staff training and supervision, secondment of staff to different programme components and development of new ways to improve delivery of clinical care.

Process evaluation

The aim of programme evaluation is to examine the clinically related procedures or activities that take place in delivering mental health services (Thornicroft and Tansella 1999). These components of care may be described in standards and clinical practice guidelines, from which quantifiable indicators of clinical practice may be derived. The main technique for process evaluation at EPPIC is the 'clinical practice review', in which clinicians look at the way services are delivered and openly discuss strategies for improvement. The aim is to evaluate aspects of care provided to patients against existing 'best practice' standards.

Practice review teams comprise three staff members – two senior staff (discipline seniors

> **Process evaluation at EPPIC**
> Questions guiding process evaluation for the Youth Access Team include:
>
> - Rate the quality of the assessments recorded in the patient notes.
> - Are any sections of the assessment form consistently missed?
> - Are diagnoses/provisional diagnoses completed?
> - Are the assessors easily identifiable?
> - How is risk assessed and managed?
> - For clients who receive a period of Youth Access Team treatment immediately following assessment, is the treatment plan documented?

- Rate the quality of the treatment plan. Is it followed?
- Are medication strategies documented?
- What happens to clients who are assessed and not accepted?
- What information is provided to the destination agency/carer?
- How is the transfer of clients within the programme managed?
- Are police used for admission or transfer?
- What is the nature of collaboration with EPPIC outpatients/inpatients/the prodrome clinic
- What documentation is provided for transfer of care?
- How are families involved in the process from intake to transfer of care?

Process audits in two other early psychosis services are outlined in the text boxes.

Process audit – example 1
The **St George Recent Onset Psychosis Intervention Project** in New South Wales, Australia, undertook a file audit of all first-episode psychosis patients attending

their service over a 4-year period (Tobin and Chen 1999, Tobin et al 1998). Adherence to early psychosis treatment guidelines was stronger during a period in which a dedicated project officer was supporting the process. However, even during that latter phase of the project, only 32% of patients had evidence of care being provided according to the guidelines.

Process audit – example 2
The **Early Psychosis Prevention and Intervention Network for Young People (EPPINY)**, in the north of Sydney, New South Wales, has developed three sets of early psychosis practice guidelines covering acute admission, medication strategies and community management. The guidelines were informed by the *Australian Clinical Guidelines for Early Psychosis* (National Early Psychosis Project Clinical Guidelines Working Party, 1998), and developed in consultation with service providers and focus groups with consumers and family members. There was also a systematic staff education programme. A checklist is being used in a retrospective 12-month audit of the medical records of 15- to 26-year-old

patients with a diagnosis of first-episode psychosis who entered services during two 6-month time periods, before and after the introduction of designated early psychosis teams. Four clinicians will examine the files of two groups of 80 patients and inter-rater reliability will be measured. There are plans to study a third cohort of patients to determine the impact of local guidelines and provision of specific staff training.

This strategy is one of three evaluation components of the EPPINY project; the others will assess clinicians' attitudes to the early intervention approach to psychosis and measure client outcomes over a 12-month period.

Enquiries:
bmoss@doh.health.nsw.gov.au or arosen@doh.health.nsw. gov.au

Outcome evaluation

Most clarificative, process and monitoring activities undertaken at EPPIC are conducted using available data and in the context of improving day-to-day practice. Outcome evaluation, however, uses more formal research techniques.

Ten programmes providing first-episode psychosis services, reviewed by Edwards et al

(2000), were contacted for details regarding their outcome evaluation protocols. The information is summarized below.

Outcome evaluation in 10 first-episode psychosis services
Evaluation domains, listed in order of how commonly they are included:

- diagnosis (common)
- symptoms – positive and negative, mood, onset (duration of untreated psychosis, duration of prodrome)
- premorbid functioning
- current functioning – social, role/occupational
- quality of life
- family and significant others – expressed emotion, social interaction, knowledge, burden
- cognition – intelligence, executive functions
- medication – nature and dose, extrapyramidal and other side effects
- life events
- personality – general, personality disorders
- physical – electrodermal activity, heart rate, blood pressure, weight/height

- treatment received/service utilization (rare)

Other domains included family or patient satisfaction, suicidality, insight, pathways to care, psychological well-being, and social networks.

An early psychosis intervention programme can use outcome data for a range of purposes, including:

- routine assessment and monitoring of outcomes at the individual client level – a process integrated into clinical practice
- aggregation for research purposes (usually without routine clinical application)
- a combination of the above

In any case, two key issues must always be considered: the definition and measurement of outcome, and the appraisal of treatment integrity.

Measuring outcome

Outcome domains such as psychotic symptomatology often receive considerable attention. However, clarification of the philosophies and aims that underpin the service are likely to indicate that other outcome domains are also relevant, such as clinical symptomatology, psychosocial functioning, disability, satisfaction with services, substance misuse and family burden. For example, EPPIC's service aims include early identification and treatment of psychotic symptoms, educating clients and families about the illness, and minimizing the impact of a psychotic episode on a young person's life. Evaluation questions to determine whether these aims have been achieved include:

- Is there a reduction in the duration of untreated psychosis for new referrals to EPPIC over time?
- Do clients and families have a greater (or more adaptive) understanding of the illness and how to manage it by the end of the treatment?
- Does quality of life improve over the course of the treatment?

It is difficult to determine which outcome measures to use if the treatment model and the underlying rationale of a service is poorly defined.

Examples of outcome evaluation in three first-episode psychosis services are described in the text boxes.

Outcome evaluation – example 1
The **Parachute Project, Sweden,** involves 17 Swedish psychiatric clinics that collect data on first-episode patients from a total population base of 1.5 million. It was established following a pilot study (Cullberg et al 2000; see Svedberg et al 2001 for further information on the historical comparison group). Participating services aim to fulfil the following six principles over a 2-year period:

- early intervention
- crisis and psychotherapeutic approach
- family approach
- continuity and easy accessibility
- lowest effective dose of antipsychotic medication
- flexible, open, home-like overnight care avoiding conventional psychiatric units if possible (at eight clinics)

A naturalistic 5-year follow up is in progress (Cullberg et al in press). Of 253 patients who entered the study (1996–1997), about 60% were prescribed antipsychotic medication, with a median dose equivalent to 1.0–2.5 mg haloperidol. Twelve-month follow-up data show significantly better improvement in the mean GAF score for the eight centres that have alternative 'crisis homes', compared with Parachute centers that have conventional inpatient care and with a prospective control group. The control group used higher doses of antipsychotic medication and had a trend towards less successful outcome on the Global Assessment of Functioning (GAF; Am Psychiatric Assoc 1987). At 12 months symptom levels did not differ between the groups. Analyses at 3 and 5 years are being carried out.

Outcome evaluation – example 2
The **Early Psychosis Outcome Evaluation System (EPOES),** Western Australia, has been devised to capture clinical outcome data. The system records clinical assessments of patients at intake, then every 6 months and at discharge. Information is obtained from case managers, clients and family members. Clinicians and support staff can produce immediate graphical representations across a range of instruments. EPOES is being used alongside usual clinical work practices in a number of Perth early psychosis programmes, enabling the capture of similar data that can be merged for comparison at a later stage.

Enquiries: neil.preston@health.wa.gov.au

Outcome evaluation – example 3

An evaluation of the **EPPIC Group Programme** has included both the processes and the outcomes (Albiston et al 1998). Patients using the service were assessed on a range of symptom and functional instruments at entry, after 6 weeks and after 6 months. All participants received comprehensive case management according to their needs. The evaluation compared 34 patients who attended the group programme and 61 who did not.

The people attending the group programme had a lower level of premorbid adjustment than the comparison group, and a trend towards a higher level of negative symptoms at baseline. However, at the 6-month follow up there were no significant differences. The evaluation concluded that involvement in the group programme may have had a positive impact on a subgroup of EPPIC patients with a poor level of premorbid adjustment, by providing a 'holding pattern' in the critical period following the onset of psychosis.

The most comprehensive EPPIC outcome project to date comprised a longitudinal naturalistic study of the effectiveness of the EPPIC model, compared with an earlier less specialized model of care (McGorry et al 1996). Chapter 5 provides details and outlines evaluation studies that are in progress.

Evaluation in practice

What information to collect is only part of any discussion about measuring outcomes. Equally important are questions about:

- identification of instruments relevant to the goals of the evaluation
- the intervals over which to collect information (e.g. standardized time intervals, episodes of care/illness, phases of illness)
- methods of data analysis
- data collection – who does it and how to integrate it into practice
- data management
- resourcing the project
- feedback to patients and staff

Treatment integrity

The experimental evaluation of multi-component treatment models is complex. An important part of the process is to evaluate the integrity of treatments – that is, the difference between what is 'promised' and what is 'delivered'. Failure to evaluate treatment integrity has two major implications:

- First, replication of methods in clinical settings is problematic or impossible (Mechanic 1996). Many studies of effectiveness and efficacy fail to adequately describe the intervention under study.
- Second, client outcomes are difficult to attribute to the interventions provided.

Details of the treatment *actually delivered* by services are essential to allow an understanding of how individual aspects of treatment, and the complex treatment model as a whole, influence patient outcome. A recent review of case management for severe mental illness concluded that, despite apparently stringent designs in most of the 75 studies, the lack of detail about the treatments provided resulted in a "limited understanding of the factors responsible for successful or unsuccessful application of these models ... [or] determinants of positive and negative outcomes" (Mueser et al 1998, p. 65). Note that another meta-analysis of case management (Ziguras and Stuart 2000) found that it led to small to moderate improvements in the effectiveness of mental health services. Assertive community treatment had some demonstrable advantages over clinical case management in reducing hospitalization.

The theoretical basis of the model and details of the treatment approach as it has evolved have been documented by EPPIC (Edwards and McGorry 1998, McGorry et al 1996). The original *EPPIC Standards of Quality in Clinical Care* (and indicators of service provision) have since been superseded by the *Australian Clinical Practice Guidelines for Early Psychosis*. Further, EPPIC Statewide Services have developed and implemented early psychosis workshops, seminars and projects throughout Victoria. The associated training materials, including an outpatient case management handbook (EPPIC 2001a), clearly document the EPPIC model with respect to a wide range of treatment issues. Documenting components of care is a good basis for ensuring fidelity but does not provide evidence of it. The second crucial aspect of evaluating treatment integrity – comparing the treatment ideal with what is actually received – is reflected in the paper by Power et al (1998, see p. 123).

Integrating programme description and evaluation

'Impact' research evaluates the influence of an entire programme and can be used to shed further light on the 'black box' of treatment (Mechanic 1996). Programme evaluation and impact evaluation can be distinguished on a number of grounds, including:

- the rationale for the activities – within-service improvement or contribution to scientific knowledge?

- facilitators – clinical staff or researchers?
- audience – programme staff or broader scientific community?
- perceived reliability of the information – 'low-grade' evaluation or 'high-grade' research?

Using evaluation data to enrich programme impact research

Strategies to clarify the integrity of treatments provided in the real-world clinical setting will depend on the nature of evaluation data collected. Interpreting the results of impact evaluation could include:

- Information on changes in service models and organizational structure, which emerges from *programme review* sessions: for example, structural organizational changes on the nature of services available to certain groups of clients (such as the availability of new interventions or the cessation of particular service modules) may be more clearly identified and understood.
- Information collected in *process evaluations*, which qualitatively document variations in service delivery: for example, a clinical practice review may indicate that a visiting registrar implemented an activity-based group that was successful for patients who were difficult to engage.

- *Monitoring data* which quantitatively document trends in service delivery: for example, monitoring data may indicate that referral and intake rates for the service have been abnormally low for some months, resulting in a fall in clinician case loads. This information may clarify the reason for temporary increases in the average number and length of contact with existing clients.

There is a growing movement to use existing clinical data to generate practice-based research (Epstein et al in press). At EPPIC, this approach was used to study the initial treatment phase of psychosis (Power et al 1998). A wide range of information including diagnosis, medication patterns and hospitalization (including seclusion, delay to admission, length of stay and readmission) were extracted from clinical records. This information was used to describe the evolution of the programme (such as sources of referrals and referral rates) and its context.

The 'big' question: does early intervention in first-episode psychosis lead to better outcomes compared to routine clinical care?

In some programmes, the impact of early intervention has been examined only by comparing outcomes before and after an intervention was introduced (e.g. Addington and Addington 2001a, Malla et al 2001 – both outlined in Chapter 5). An advance on this design is the use of historical controls for comparison purposes (e.g. McGorry et al 1996; Parachute Project – described on page 120). The historical control group design has weaknesses as there may be factors other than the intervention that affect the outcome, such as variance in population and treatment over time.

The alternative is to use concurrent controls, for example patients assessed in nearby catchment areas during the same follow-up period (e.g. EPPIC Statewide Services *Early Psychosis Projects*; TIPS – described in Chapter 5; Catts et al in press). However, cohorts may differ in a range of variables such as socioeconomic status. A more sophisticated design is the randomized controlled trial, which is being attempted in the UK (see text box). This is ideally achieved in a new service, to avoid the difficulties of services withholding apparently optimal treatments from a proportion of clients. However, the disadvantage is that a new service may not have sufficient time to focus on the impact of different interventions, and the apparent effect of interventions may be underestimated because of other factors such as clinical skill development and high treatment integrity. Additionally, negative feelings of staff in comparative programmes is likely, as one

programme is perceived as an inferior control and the other programme is perceived as having additional expertise or resources (Catts et al in press). There is need for a range of designs that will shed light on different aspects of early intervention in psychotic disorders.

Randomized controlled trial of early intervention, UK

In Lambeth, a multicultural, inner-city London Borough, the South London and Maudsley Trust is developing a new early intervention program. The **Lambeth Early Onset (LEO) service** (www.slam.nhs.uk) includes a specialised 18-bed inpatient unit and a community-based assertive outreach service which is being evaluated in a randomized controlled trial (Garety and Jolley 2000). Patients are eligible for the study if they are aged 16–40 years, live in the catchment area (population approximately 270 000), and present with a first or second episode of a schizophrenia spectrum disorder. Randomization occurs at the point of referral to psychiatric services; consent is sought for research ratings and for postrandomization follow-up. The treatment package includes:

- psychological interventions
- family work
- facilitation of access to education and employment
- service user involvement
- integrated care for patients with dual diagnoses
- optimal low-dose antipsychotic treatment

The control group receives standard care as delivered through pre-existing teams. Clinical and social outcomes are assessed within a week of allocation and at 6 and 18 months.

Evaluation and quality officer

Without dedicated funding for evaluation, services may lack:

- staff support for collection and analysis of data
- expertise, interest or time on the part of clinicians
- systems for ongoing monitoring (e.g. routine patient-level outcome data, serious incidents, key performance indicators, quality assurance) (Burgess and Pirkis 1999)

In the busy clinical environment, it is easy to consider evaluation a non-essential activity and decision makers may be reluctant to dedicate the funds required to sustain routine evaluation. Funders and providers of mental health services must both view evaluation as an integral component of the mental health service structure.

Services may find that costs of evaluation can be managed by building evaluation tasks into existing positions, especially at an administrative level. The full costs of the implementation and ongoing support for comprehensive service evaluation should not be underestimated. In Australia, there is a preference for evaluation to be conducted by an external independent evaluator or team. Despite the obvious advantages of such an approach, this may operate as a disincentive to build evaluation roles into the routine service system.

> **Suggested responsibilities duties of an evaluation and quality officer**
> - develop, implement and actively participate in the delivery of evaluation and quality assurance activities
> - provide support, guidance and assistance to staff regarding evaluation issues
> - undertake 'mini' evaluation/research projects

- coordinate data management systems for clinical subprogrammes and produce summaries of clinical data
- in consultation with the programme executive, prepare briefing documents, service reports and resource materials
- develop funding submissions

The concept of specialized services for first-episode psychosis is relatively new. Continued development and expansion of such services will depend on the benefits and costs being determined, and then communicated clearly to all stakeholders.

Real-world considerations

Investment in new and better treatments must continue, but we must learn to deliver them effectively in real-world settings. (McGorry 2000, p. 22)

Although vision is important for initiating change, it is not enough to organize and maintain a system of care. Vision must be translated into practical strategies. (Rosen et al 1997, p. 29)

There are likely to be numerous decision points and obstacles when implementing early intervention in psychosis. This chapter provides 'food for thought', tackling some of the common queries, challenges and organizational issues. It concludes with an example of a process for implementing a focus on early intervention services.

Service model

Ethics of intervention in the prepsychotic phase

A range of ethical issues needs to be considered in relation to the prepsychotic phase (McGorry et al 2001c, Rosen 2000).

Caution is required to avoid unnecessary stigmatization of non-psychotic individuals as 'prepsychotic'. Preventive treatment may be given to individuals who would have had a good prognosis if left untreated, or who would not have developed psychosis at all (i.e. false positives). The young people seen at the Melbourne PACE clinic (see Chapter 2) are a help-seeking clinical population who are distressed and disabled by their symptoms, regardless of their final diagnosis. Research is urgently required to clarify optimal treatments to alleviate their distress and disability, and to reduce their risk of subsequent psychosis. In the interim, however, there is a need for a clinical response from community mental health services and primary care in order to relieve their distress and disability. An offer of initial problem-focused psychosocial treatment including cognitive therapies, with or without symptom-based drug treatments, seems justifiable as a component of a low-stigma youth-oriented mental health service.

Many clinicians will be reluctant to prescribe antipsychotic medications for high-risk patients who do not yet have clear psychotic symptoms. Patients themselves may resist taking antipsychotic medications (and suffering the potential adverse side effects) just to reduce the possibility of crossing a theoretical threshold to psychosis. Caution is appropriate at this stage, until results emerge from current research to define those most at risk and the benefits of intervention.

There is little point in early detection if best-practise treatments are not used following the onset of psychosis. In our opinion, a research clinic for high-risk individuals should be developed only within the context of a specialized first-episode psychosis service. Access to follow up for distressed help-seekers who do not meet the criteria for the research clinic is also needed, and will require good links with primary health workers.

Client and family involvement

Provision for client involvement in an early psychosis service needs to recognize that these individuals and their families have different perspectives to those experiencing chronic mental illnesses. Their role needs to reflect these differences, rather than following a standard model of peer participation. Many people who experience early psychosis are relatively brief users of mental health services and may not find a peer participation role relevant or meaningful. Others struggle to cope with the experience of the illness and its treatment, and consequently may find it difficult to contribute. Nevertheless, it is essential to ensure that there is a strong client influence on the service because this maximizes respect for service users and enhances the ambience and quality of care. Consulting with recent 'graduates' of early treatment may introduce some protective 'distance' from the experience of illness and the distress of the acute phase of psychosis. Whatever mechanisms are used for recruitment, a positive policy towards people with experience of mental health problems should be encouraged (May 2000).

Families and friends should also be involved in the development of early psychosis services. Public lectures on early psychosis, advertised in newspapers or other media, are one way of gaining their interest, and members of local schizophrenia family support associations can be invited. Within a psychiatric service, invitations can be circulated to family members, seeking those who are willing to participate in an early psychosis advisory group or a first-episode self-support parent group. When establishing support groups it can be useful for a staff member to fill a dual role as facilitator and the spokesperson for programme management (Catts et al in press).

Examples of consumer and family participation are outlined in the text boxes.

Consumer involvement

The **Early Psychosis Intervention Program (EPIP)**, in Liverpool, New South Wales, Australia, has developed a youth consumer group in which up to five paid youth consumers and a staff member meet fortnightly to discuss, plan and undertake projects.

There is also a monthly meeting with director of the programme to discuss provision of services to young people with psychosis. Activities include:

- submitting a grant to develop a youth consumer training programme
- identifying a need for information sheets relevant to youth experiencing psychosis in the sector – suggesting the main themes and surveying available material
- employing a client on a part-time basis to support young people who require admission to the adult inpatient unit
- undertaking site visits to other early intervention programmes to investigate service provision options

---

Family involvement

"My son entered the PEPP Program, Ontario, Canada [see Chapter 5] in November 1997, at the age of 17. During those early days my husband and I came to know a handful of parents who were in similar circumstances. Shortly after, there was an immediate concern that cuts could be made to PEPP staff as provincial government funds were not allocated as mandated. Our small group of parents mobilised quickly, petitioned the powers that be and, within a matter of weeks, were successful that seeing funds were put in place!

"We continued meeting together over coffee to discuss our day-to-day challenges and concerns. It was such a relief to be able to talk about the illness with people who knew exactly what we were feeling. Although we did not know it at the time, the seeds of a parent group were being planted. In early June of 1998, our little coffee group posted invitations, at the clinic and on the hospital unit, for other PEPP parents to join us. The response was heart-warming. Now in our third year our PEPP Parent Support Group numbers more than 30 families!

"We meet at the clinic the third Wednesday of each month from 7.00–10.00 pm. Our primary goals are peer support and advocacy for our children. However there are those of us who have moved beyond the 'reactive' phase and are now assuming a more 'proactive' role. We attend seminars, workshops, conferences etc here in London and throughout the province, speaking to high school and university classes, participate and help organise the annual public forums, assist with PEPP's early case detection campaign, conduct bake and craft sales, partner with PEPP to stage the annual dinner/dance/fund-raiser etc. We have also had input with the publication of a newsletter aptly named 'Family to Family' for first episode psychosis families (www.cmha.ca) which we hope will service to link clinics and family groups across Canada. I was thrilled to be able to represent the PEPP Parent Support Group at last year's IEPA Conference in New York City."

PEPP Parent Support Group member

The video *One Day at a Time* (www.cmha.ca) provides an overview of the rationale and development of the PEPP Parent Support Group and may be a useful resource to assist establishment of similar groups.

Specialist versus generalist models

We take for granted that specialised teams will deliver specialised treatment for virtually all serious conditions such as burns, cardiac disorders, or children's cancer. Schizophrenia is the most costly disorder to treat ... The only way to improve the standard of care and reduce this cost is by incorporating the many recent innovations in treatment. This can only be done by specialist training and specialist service delivery. (Catts et al in press).

Proponents of specialist models of service delivery (for example, Catts et al in press) and proponents of generalist models (for example, Tobin and Chen 1999) each advance strong arguments. 'Hybrid' models (*IRIS Clinical Guidelines and Service Frameworks*, pp. 33–35; see Chapter 5) are located between these two options. On examining the 'pros' and 'cons' of each model, summarized in Table 8.1, a generalist model seems difficult to sustain in the long term. Attempts to incorporate key elements of specialist services into mainstream mental health services requires at least a dedicated project worker or clinical specialist, ideally an experienced and credible senior clinician, whose stated duties include:

- planning and coordination of early psychosis initiatives
- provision of staff education and clinical supervision in early psychosis
- development of local first-episode psychosis treatment protocols
- implementation of a system to monitor and review first-episode psychosis patients, including service entry and exit
- undertaking early psychosis clinical services (e.g. family work, group work)

- establishing links with relevant psychiatric disability support services
- provision of community development activities in consultation with primary care teams
- distribution of early psychosis resource materials
- overseeing evaluation and research

Middle managers may have concerns that encouragement of early intervention will lead to staff being overwhelmed by new cases. They may also be aware that an early intervention approach is more resource intensive, with additional time and input required to maximize recovery as well as provide optimal assistance to the family. Dedicated resources for an early psychosis service will help to define the expectations of all concerned.

Provision of special care to early psychosis patients in an inpatient setting with a mixed patient group is a challenging, if not impossible, task. There are a number of early psychosis inpatient units which focus on early and/or late recovery, for example the Adolescent Clinic at Amsterdam Medical Clinic in The Netherlands and the Berne First Episode Psychosis Program in Switzerland (see Edwards et al 2000 for descriptions of these two services) and EIS in Birmingham (see Chapter 5). Some offer long inpatient stays (for 6 months or more) and operate on psychodynamic/rehabilitation principles (e.g. the Clinic for Child and Adolescent Psychiatry at Olgahospital Stuttgart,

Table 8.1
Pros and cons of specialist and generalist early psychosis service models

Specialist

Pros

- Separation from patients with more established illnesses
- Creation of youth friendly environment
- Separate team structure allows the fostering of a team philosophy and undertaking of developmental activities within a supportive atmosphere
- Dedicated intake service provides the opportunity to assess barriers to young people seeking referral and to design procedures that are 'user friendly' to referring agents
- Improves client detection rates, client retention rates, and client and carer engagement
- Research opportunities
- Dedicated clinical leadership usually inherent

Cons

- Requires supplementary resources
- Proliferation of subspecialist programmes for every special needs groups
- Loss of quality personnel and expertise progressively from generalist services
- A 'stand-alone' service could become isolated and have difficulties in providing after-hours cover and ensuring continuity of care
- Staff may become overloaded if insufficient resources or poor exit criteria

Generalist

Pros

- Creation of an environment of awareness of early intervention and awareness among all staff
- Provides a framework for professional development and morale enhancement

Cons

- Difficult to incorporate new ideas into routine clinical practice in routine mental health settings due to poor morale and generic nature of the service
- Early psychosis initiatives are often considered additional to core business/chronic schizophrenia, and is difficult to sustain and evaluate in the context of high case loads
- Difficult to survive when resources are tight – easy dismantle specialist foci within service reconfiguration
- Cultural ingredients (e.g. egalitarianism and optimism – see text) difficult to foster

Germany; Ulleval Hospital in Oslo, Sweden; U7 at Sct. Hans Hospital, Copenhagen, Denmark). However, there are few examples of specialized inpatient services providing care during the acute phase which are integrated with outpatient services (e.g. EPPIC and PEPP – see Chapter 5; LEO – see Chapter 7; First Episode Psychosis Program, Toronto – outlined in the text box).

Integrated care
The **First Episode Psychosis Program at the Centre for Addiction and Mental Health, University of Toronto, Ontario, Canada,** was developed in 1992 as an integrated inpatient–outpatient programme. It has a 12-bed inpatient unit devoted to the care of patients experiencing a first episode of non-affective psychosis. The programme has access to additional resources such as a high school programme for individuals with mental illness (operated by the local board of education) and a psychosocial clubhouse for chronically mentally ill patients (located in a nearby house), which has evolved to meet the needs of first-episode psychosis patients. Plans for a specialized learning centre are underway.

Currently 150 new cases are accepted each year and the standing case load is 200 individuals. The programme has recently received funding from the Government of Ontario to implement a mobile assessment and treatment team. With added resources, it is expected that there will be capacity to assess approximately 400 new cases of affective and non-affective psychosis each year from metropolitan Toronto (population 4 million). The first-episode service has become the heart of schizophrenia research at the University of Toronto, with a focus on the neurobiological basis of schizophrenia and its pharmacological treatment (Kapur et al 1999, 2000, Zipursky et al 1998, 2001).

Enquiries: robert_zipursky@ camh.net

Challenges
Where is the evidence?

The practitioner must choose. Shall he remain on the high ground where he can solve relatively unimportant problems according to prevailing standards of rigour, or shall he descend to the swamp of important problems and non-rigorous enquiry? (Schön 1990, p. 3)

Strictly speaking, randomised controlled trials are still needed to confirm the effectiveness of early detection and intervention services. However, the testimony of patients and families, non-randomised evaluations of services such as those provided by the Early Psychosis Prevention and Intervention Centre services and obvious validity or common sense supports their wider introduction. (Lewis and Drake 2001, p. 142)

Excessive negativity or caution on the basis that the relevant evidence has not yet emerged could be harmful to the process of collecting sufficient data. There is a danger of 'killing off' the enthusiasm for this focus in psychiatry before the evidence fully emerges. As noted by Larsen et al (2001), drawing parallels with the early treatment of rheumatoid arthritis (Scott and Huskisson 1992), a shortening of the time for which a patient is overtly psychotic is obviously beneficial, *even if* the long-term outcomes are not changed. It seems likely that the quality of life during the first years of illness will be improved when early treatment is achieved, simply by reducing the time that a patient is symptomatic. The burden of disease can be reduced even if final outcomes are not substantially altered.

Thornicroft and Tansella (1999) argue that

the technical solutions of evidence based medicine should not be used alone to respond adequately to complex planning choices. Rather, the evidence base should be counter-balanced by a principal ethical base, and in our view the primary responsibility for introducing clinical value to these decisions lies with clinicians (p. 141).

The widespread introduction of case management in mental health services prior to demonstrable effectiveness (Mueser et al 1998, Ziguras and Stuart 2000) is one example of a practice becoming established before evidence was available for its efficacy. The written statement of principles produced by an early psychosis service (see Chapter 6, Step 1) should reflect a sound ethical base, allowing development of a service in which scientific evidence can be collected over a period of years. Most service reforms are driven by sociopolitical factors and, at best, based on perceived gaps and deficiencies that cannot be ignored, because of political pressure and community needs.

Funding arguments

Resources for mental health services are finite and generally scarce. Even when resources are abundant it seems to be common to provide primarily for patients who have established disorders and to continue to configure services to cater for such patients. This has also been a problem in the mainstream health system, where expensive high-technology interventions are delivered to patients with end-stage chronic disease, while preventive interventions in the earlier stages of illness fail to receive adequate support. Older psychotic patients with significant disability tend – not unreasonably – to be seen as 'more severe', and their characteristics contribute almost exclusively to the definition of 'serious mental illness'. A more dynamic understanding of 'disorder' enables the potential for prevention to be appreciated more fully. Giving priority to established cases ignores the chance to reduce the size of this group in the future, and to reduce the need for belated 'rescue' or palliative therapies. For example, family interventions initiated several years after the onset of illness, against a background of neglect, detachment or high expressed emotion, are almost certainly less cost effective than earlier interventions. There will be a lag between initiating early services and reaping the potential financial benefits, so a certain amount of vision in service planning and longer-term budget cycles may be required.

Arguments have been advanced that mental health resources should be directed at more prevalent disorders such as anxiety and depression. However, the quality of life of many people with psychotic disorders remains very poor (Jablensky et al 1999) and there is enormous scope for improvement in the treatment of these serious, but lower-prevalence, disorders.

Health care system

In some health services, inpatient and outpatient care are managed in different structures. This division works against the development of creative community-focused services and integrated service systems for early psychosis patients. In the model of care provided for first-episode psychosis in EPPIC's current catchment area, but prior to the formation of EPPIC, this division also worked against shortening the duration of untreated psychosis (McGorry et al 1996). The way in which services were delivered in Victoria changed dramatically in the early 1990s, blurring the barriers between inpatient and outpatient services.

Providing care for first-episode patients within the USA managed care environment is particularly challenging. Because consensus about the appropriate treatment of first-episode psychosis is still emerging, controversy can arise between the managed care funder and the providers about what kind of treatment is necessary. The onus is on clinicians and academics

to educate managed care organisations, legislators, and the public at large about standards of care for serious illnesses so that arbitrary standards are not adopted solely on the basis of cost (Jarskog et al 2000, p. 883).

Managed care and detection of early psychosis

The **Portland Identification and Early Referral Project (PIER)**, Maine, USA, is a pilot project funded by a private foundation. Greater Portland (population 240 000) has a recently established and widespread interest in early intervention. Support from key representatives of the target populations, leaders of professional groups, and consumer and advocacy organizations was readily secured in developing the funding submission. Primary care physicians are involved in a not-for-profit managed care system that places them at financial risk if one of their enrolled patients becomes psychotic and is hospitalized. The PIER Project offers the possibility of arresting that process. It has been proposed that prodromal schizophrenia be added to the list of disorders covered by the managed care system.

The first phase of PIER targets physicians, schools and colleges, social workers, guidance counsellors, high school nurses, police and others likely to encounter young people at risk of psychosis. The second phase is a public education campaign (assisted by a public relations firm) that educates families, young people and the general population about early warning signs of psychosis. Phase three will establish an assessment and treatment service that will identify individuals aged 12–30 years who are at substantial risk of psychosis or are already ill, and provide medication, family intervention and education.

Enquiries: mcfarw@mmc.org

Managed care and early assessment

The **Early Assessment and Support Team (EAST)** is an initiative of the Mid-Valley Behavioral Care Network (MVBCN) in Salem, Oregon, USA. The aim of EAST is to identify and support individuals aged 15–30 years who have first-episode psychosis. The MVBCN is a managed mental health care entity responsible for Medicaid-funded services in five counties (population 600 000) which is able to reinvest its resources proactively to prevent future disability. The project encourages investment by private health care insurers.

The EAST team includes a coordinator and part-time psychiatrist, and part-time staff from nine agencies. Community education is provided to doctors, school officials, clergy, law enforcement and other professionals, as well as the media and general public. Referrals are made directly to team members or through a centralized phone number. The approach combines psychoeducation, cognitive therapy, supportive case management, family support and education, and a low-dose medication protocol.

Enquiries: kathys@mvbcn.org

Early psychosis services in developing countries

Three-quarters of the world's population lives in developing countries, where there is a need to develop indigenous mental health programmes that target specific areas (Rahman et al 2000). Challenges include:

- the low priority given to health and education
- the needs of local populations exceeding available resources
- the scarcity of trained mental health professionals, with a need for involvement of non-specialized health workers
- lack of infrastructure
- developing sustainable programmes (e.g. will access to medication be available beyond a clinical trial?)
- the stigma attached to mental disorders – there is a need to educate extended families
- religious and cultural issues concerning the meaning of mental illness

Organizational issues

Egalitarian culture

Early psychosis services seem to flourish when they are developed in an egalitarian environment that allows sharing of ideas between staff members and the application of management principles that encourage discussion and common ownership of the service's policies and principles. Our interpretation of this phenomenon is that:

- Adolescents struggle with issues of independence and psychosis is a blow to self-esteem.
- respect for the patient's retained decision-making capacity can have a restorative function.
- Relationships between leaders and staff in an early psychosis service should reflect ideal clinician–patient interactions that respect independence and decision-making.

Articulating a philosophy is a component of an egalitarian culture in which patients, families and staff have a right to understand plans and expectations, and clinicians have a responsibility to communicate vision and explanations of elements of care.

Leadership

A 'special focus' service will benefit if it is established with an emphasis on the programme that is to be provided, rather than the disciplines that will operate it. The existence of a team leader (ideally, an experienced senior clinician) with a clear statement of goals and authority to take action can help focus resources on particular tasks. Specialist expertise from a number of disciplines can then be recruited to the programme and deployed within a multidisciplinary team. It is important that the team leader mandates others to undertake leadership roles, including presenting the service at key forums, to deliberately "broaden the leadership base" (Rosen et al 1997, p. 29). Working parties and committees should have clearly identified convenors, operate with terms of reference and appoint chairpersons. Managers and funding authorities need to allocate resources so that coordination and effective clinical leadership can occur.

Optimism

Embracing an optimistic approach, and communicating optimism to all involved, is a crucial factor in successfully implementing change. Many staff are aware of the danger of 'rescue fantasies', but pessimism about the management of schizophrenia has traditionally been extreme and a substantial degree of realistic optimism is justified. An optimistic approach in early psychosis breeds and sustains morale in a service. The optimism is readily communicated to the patients and this attitude not only promotes recovery but may potentially lead to improved outcomes, including reduced suicide rates.

Programme survival

A healthy organization needs to be alert for possible improvement and positive change. Such change should, however, occur against a background of stable organizational values and a clearly defined and stable 'mission'. Increasing exposure and legitimacy is an important factor in programme survival, so publicity and obtaining awards and grants should be encouraged (Rosen et al 1997). Links with local, national and international communities at the level of service delivery, policy development and academic activities, for example through attendance and presentations at conferences, is important. Developing a web site (see text box) and publishing descriptive service accounts and research findings are other means of communicating with the wider community. A focus on early psychosis needs to be established as the accepted standard, and translation into government policy is the goal. (See Chapter 5 for policy examples in Australia and the UK.)

Developing a web site

The internet is a powerful communication tool, and web sites are a relatively straightforward way for services to communicate with clients, colleagues and the general public. Issues to be considered in establishing a web site include:

- What information do you wish to convey? Do you want to share information on your research, describe your clinical services, put a face to your staff, list current resources, advise people how to refer to your service, provide support online for families and clients, recruit staff, or strengthen national networks? Is the site an opportunity to set a corporate identity for your service and create 'brand' recognition that adds to other communication strategies?

- Who is the target audience? It may be people who are referring patients to the service, clinicians working in the same field nationally or internationally, or the general public in your region.
- What information does your target audience require? Pre-testing the content can be valuable in refining the content.
- Who will construct and maintain the site? Will technical problems be resolved quickly so that the site is reliable?

Practical suggestions include:

- Use key messages as banners on the home page.
- Check your site for readability and ease of navigation among your target audience.
- When designing the site, take account of the hardware and software your users are likely to have.
- Keep the text succinct, pithy and fairly specific. Longer articles or publications can be added in a format that is downloaded by the user.
- Check with other sites first, if you are intending to include them as links.

- Provide accurate and up-to-date e-mail addresses for contact, and ensure that e-mails obtained through the site are answered promptly.
- Mark each page with the date it was last updated.
- Add a disclaimer or a 'statement of intent' to describe the purpose and limitations of the site.
- If the site provides on-line counselling, accepts referrals or even has chat groups targeted at people experiencing psychosis, take note of the duty of care associated with such a service.

Professional development

Training, education, and consultation are necessary to bring about change within a service and to successfully develop a new approach. Investment in staff development is one of the most important factors to consider when establishing an early psychosis service. Techniques can range from distribution of academic papers to more comprehensive programmes.

Training

Consideration should be given to the format and content used by trainers. It is essential to match the topic and pitch of the information to the participants' needs. For example, in a large group with little background in early psychosis, it will be important to discuss the philosophical underpinning of the preventive approach and the rationale for early intervention before covering issues such as at-risk mental states and assessment. With a group with some background in the area, or with particular professional skills (such as psychotherapy), it will be possible to address specific areas within the field such as cognitive–behavioural therapy or family work.

Training in the early stages normally focuses on attitudes and knowledge, which might be approached through a series of lectures or 1- or 2-day workshops. At a later stage the focus can move to advanced skills that will require more intensive input and will possibly include supervision arrangements.

Training pack

The *Early Psychosis Training Pack* (McGorry and Edwards 1997) was established on a train-the-trainer model for mental health workers, and each module contains numerous vignettes and teaching exercises (download via www.epic.org.au or www.futur.com). The kit is available in Dutch, German, and Spanish. Austrian and Portuguese translations are in progress. The German, Austrian and Portuguese modules include PowerPoint presentations. The *Training Pack* has also been reworked into a format for general practitioners, available in French (there are also plans to consider a Flemish version). Spanish copies can be obtained by contacting psiquiat@ipmq.higgm.es. The other translations can be downloaded from www.psychiatry24x7.com.

It is useful for the training group to reconvene regularly to discuss how its members have been able to implement their new skills and knowledge, and to use the process of group discussions to work through challenges and dilemmas. One approach is to form a peer support/supervision group or a mentor/buddy system in which two or three participants support one another in the early stages after a formal training programme as they begin to use their new skills. Distance learning through videoconferencing, webcasting, internet-based packages, or using video, audiotape and CD-ROM materials can also be effective. More extended postgraduate education can be provided through creating modules within broader courses and programmes. Written materials in the form of key references, handouts, clinical guides, workbooks and practice manuals can be used to enhance knowledge independently of workshops or lectures.

Examples of postgraduate education with a focus on early psychosis

- The Graduate Diploma in Mental Health Sciences (Young People's Mental Health) is provided through distance education by EPPIC and the Department of Psychiatry, University of Melbourne, Australia (www.eppic.org.au).
- The Education and Training Programme, developed by the SAFE project (see Chapter 7) to enhance the basic skill level of clinicians working with early psychosis in rural areas, has been endorsed by the New South Wales Institute of Psychiatry.

Site visits and expert speakers

Site visits can allow clinicians to exchange expertise, experience and challenges. Many of the services described in this book are receptive to requests for site visits and some have organized regional or national conferences on early psychosis. Such visits and conferences can be important in influencing policy makers and clinicians, and offer the host service an opportunity to access expert speakers for the benefit of their own staff.

Exposure to early psychosis conferences will assist in decisions with regard to choosing the 'right' speakers for a service activity.

Consultation

Consultation promotes a collaborative partnership to identify solutions to problems and challenges. Mental health consultation can involve:

- client-centred case consultation, relating to the management of a particular case or group of cases
- consultee-centred consultation, which aims to help the consultee to improve knowledge and skills
- programme-centred consultation, which aims to improve planning, administration and programme development

It is necessary for the individuals providing the consultation to be closely allied with a clinical setting, and to draw on the experience of clinicians at that service. The drawback of this model is that it needs a 'home base' from which trainers and experts can be drawn, and this base must be able to fund and resource such activities. A mandate from the purchasers of services, together with appropriate funding, is an essential foundation. A broader range of activities can be funded on a fee-for-service basis.

The EPPIC *Early Psychosis Projects*: a model for supporting new service initiatives

The project has been enthusiastically embraced by staff and has effected major change in culture and practice. (Service manager, Mental Health Service)

The Statewide Services (see Chapter 5) subprogramme of EPPIC undertook Early Psychosis Projects involving intense work with an adult mental health service for 6 months, leaving structures in place to develop and promote best practice in early psychosis. Six early psychosis projects have been completed in metropolitan Melbourne and rural areas of Victoria. The aims of the projects reflect local priorities and resources, but usually include:

- ensuring the early identification and treatment of the primary symptoms of psychotic illness, by improving access to specialized services
- minimizing secondary morbidity, disruption in social and vocational functioning and carer burden
- promoting well-being among family members

Each project involves the formation of:

- a *Steering Group* to oversee and support

the development and implementation of the project and ensure appropriate evaluation, comprising senior management from the relevant department of psychiatry or mental health service, EPPIC Statewide Services and the state government branch of the psychiatric services

- a *Clinicians' Group* to address day-to-day issues and consider the key activities in detail, comprising discipline seniors, subprogramme managers of the adult mental health service and the local child and adolescent mental health service, other interested local clinicians, and representatives of the psychiatric disability support services
- *working parties.*

Individual working parties typically address the following issues:

- *community development and education* – development of local community education campaigns; information and training sessions for primary care workers and general practitioners; education of other service providers on the special issues and needs of patients with early psychosis
- *professional education and training* – seminars and education sessions for local mental health professionals on best practice in early psychosis; development of a peer supervision group to focus on the psychological needs of young people

recovering from psychosis; and circulation of relevant early psychosis literature

- *clinical practice* – development of strategies for local interpretation and implementation of *The Australian Clinical Guidelines for First-Episode Psychosis*; development of protocols to facilitate service access and minimize trauma; and facilitation of secondary consultation as required
- *family work* – development of protocols for optimal management of the families of clients with early psychosis; and development of information/support groups/seminars for the families of clients with early psychosis
- *group activities* – working with psychiatric disability support services to develop group activities appropriate for age and phase of illness

Early Psychosis Projects have operated in response to recognition by services that they should focus on early intervention as well as the more traditional demands of chronic psychotic disorders. Previously many individuals with first-episode psychosis were not accepted by these services, which assumed they required less intensive services and might be managed by private psychiatrists or other providers. Other concerns of the services involved fear of increasing workloads in already busy settings. One of the results of the *Early Psychosis Projects* has been the development of a more therapeutic approach to patients with schizophrenia, especially family psychoeducation and peer support, and more uniform provision of low-dose and novel antipsychotics. Site visits and workshops provided by the EPPIC Statewide Services provided an environment of knowledge sharing, which fed and sustained the momentum. Formal evaluation has occurred in two regions in which the Projects operated (Krstev et al 2001b).

Early psychosis work was recognised as important by both management and the clinical team . . . This made it easier to be involved in projects, such as group work, which are sometimes seen as additional to core business. Enthusiasm contributes to staff being willing to go the 'extra mile' in terms of service delivery. (Case manager, Mental Health Service)

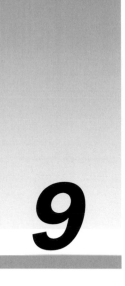

Draft consensus statement – principles and practice in early psychosis

9

Introduction

The delivery of care in early psychosis is often delayed, piecemeal and alienating to patients and families. Patients usually have to cross a high threshold of disturbance and risk to gain access to treatment, and have to demonstrate a persistent and pervasive level of disability (or activity limitation/participation restriction) to 'earn' the right to continuing care. Treatment models are geared to the needs of older patients with chronic conditions, reinforcing the pessimism inherent in the concept of schizophrenia. Community ignorance, stigma (operating in the larger community and within mental health services), poor mental health literacy, and the isolation of psychiatry from the rest of medicine and health care add to the obstacles to reforming systems to focus on early intervention.

A special focus on the early phases of psychotic disorders is justified on three major grounds:

- The clinical care of people with first-episode psychosis is often delayed or inadequate, and sometimes crude or harmful. Some people never receive treatment.

- Increasing evidence suggests there are major opportunities for effective secondary prevention, which could substantially lower the mortality and morbidity associated with these disorders.
- Epidemiological, neurobiological and psychosocial study of early psychosis may facilitate early intervention and secondary prevention, and enable superior treatment.

There are three targets for preventive interventions in early psychosis:

- The prepsychotic phase is often prolonged and characterized by subtle and confusing symptoms. Much of the disability associated with the psychotic disorders is established and accumulates in this phase.
- The period of untreated psychosis is a risk factor for a poor outcome. It has many determinants, but there is potential for intervention within communities to reduce the duration of untreated psychosis and the distress, risk and disability associated with untreated psychosis.
- The first psychotic episode and the critical period of the early years following initial diagnosis deserves optimal, comprehensive and phase-specific treatment with continuity of care guaranteed.

This draft consensus statement identifies key principles in addressing current deficiencies for preventive intervention and proposes

strategies to enhance clinical care. The statement has been developed with input from the 26 invited international consultants who gave feedback by the publication deadline. The draft is published here with the aim of encouraging further discussion. Ratification will be sought by the executive of the International Early Psychosis Association and the final consensus statement will be presented at the Third International Conference on Early Psychosis to be held in Copenhagen, September 2002.

General statements

- Early identification of people in the earliest phases of psychotic disorders combined with optimal treatment is likely to reduce the burden of disease. Early treatment of active psychosis is beneficial in its own right, but the possibility exists that it will also improve long-term outcomes and reduce the prevalence of psychotic disorders.
- Community-wide education should be encouraged to ensure that the public has a better understanding of the onset of psychotic disorders and how to obtain effective advice, treatment and support.
- Phase-specific programmes of care, which also take into account that the majority of patients with early psychosis are young, should be developed and evaluated.
- Pharmacological treatments should be

introduced with great care in drug-naive patients, with an over-riding principle of doing the least harm while aiming for the maximum benefit. This will involve the use of the minimum effective dose of atypical or second-generation antipsychotics wherever possible, consistent with the recommendations of the World Psychiatric Association. If typical or first-generation antipsychotics cannot be avoided, which is the situation at present in developing countries, then they should be used judiciously and at very low doses.

- Psychosocial interventions have a fundamental place in early treatment, providing a humane basis for continuing care, preventing or resolving secondary consequences of the psychosis, and promoting recovery. Enhancement of professional skills and encouragement of psychosocial interventions by funding bodies are essential.

- Priority should be given to research on representative early psychosis populations to obtain a deeper understanding of the processes associated with the onset of psychosis.

- Consumers and families need to be engaged as partners in developing better treatments and with the aim of validating their experiences of early psychosis.

The prepsychotic period

Background

The prepsychotic period can be divided into two phases:

- The *premorbid phase* is the period during childhood and usually at least part of adolescence in which emotional, cognitive and behavioural functioning are not impaired.

- The *prodromal period* or symptomatic 'at-risk mental state' is usually characterized by a sustained and clinically important deviation from the premorbid level of experience and behaviour. The term 'at-risk mental state' refers to phenomenology and behaviour irrespective of the outcome.

Clinical guidelines

- The possibility of a psychotic disorder should be carefully considered in a young person who is becoming more socially withdrawn, performing worse for a sustained period at school or at work, or who is becoming more distressed or agitated yet unable to explain why.

- Some young people are at very high risk and meet the criteria for having an at-risk mental state. Criteria include:
  - subthreshold positive symptoms that are not severe or persistent enough to meet criteria sufficient for a diagnosis

of a DSM-IV/ICD-10 psychotic disorder other than 'Brief Psychotic Disorder', or

– a family history of psychotic disorder or schizotypal disorder in a first-degree relative plus a significant, persistent but non-specific decline in psychosocial functioning within the past year or so

- If young people with an at-risk mental state are actively seeking help for the distress and disability associated with their symptoms, they need to be:

  – engaged and assessed

  – offered regular monitoring of mental state and offered support

  – offered specific treatment for syndromes such as depression, anxiety or substance misuse, and assistance with problem areas such as interpersonal, vocational and family stress if present

  – provided with psychoeducation and encouraged to develop coping skills for subthreshold psychotic symptoms

  – offered family education and support

  – provided information in a flexible, careful and clear way about risks for mental disorders as well as about existing syndromes

- Such care can be carried out in a low-stigma environment such as home, primary care or youth friendly office-based setting.

- Antipsychotic medications are not usually indicated unless the person meets criteria for a DSM-IV/ICD-10 psychotic disorder. Exceptions should be considered when rapid deterioration is occurring; severe suicidal risk is present and treatment of any depression had proved ineffective; or aggression or hostility are increasing and pose a risk to others. If antipsychotics are considered, ideally atypical medications should be used in low doses and considered as a 'therapeutic trial' for a limited period. If there is benefit and resolution of symptoms after 6 weeks, the medication may be continued with the patient's consent for a further 6 months to 2 years, following explanation of risks and benefits. After this period, a gradual attempt to withdraw the medication should be made if the patient agrees and there has been a good recovery. If the patient has not responded to one atypical antipsychotic, another may be tried if the above indications still exist.

- If young people with an at-risk mental state are not seeking help, then regular contact with family members or friends may be an appropriate strategy.

- The evidence of effectiveness of treatments aimed specifically at reducing the risk of transition psychosis (e.g. cognitive and family therapy, antipsychotic medication or experimental neuroprotective drug strategies) remains preliminary. More data are required and the risk–benefit ratio of various interventions needs to be determined.

Research

- There should be better characterization of the process of transition to prodrome or at-risk mental state to frank psychosis at phenomenological, psychosocial and neurobiological levels.
- Further research is needed to determine which treatment strategies may be effective in reducing the burden of symptoms and disability in at-risk mental states, and in reducing the risk of progression to a psychotic disorder.
- Such research must meet the highest ethical standards applicable to all medical research. Patients must give genuine informed consent and be free to withdraw from research at any time. Non-participation in research must not affect access to appropriate clinical care.
- Research should be led or heavily informed by local clinicians and researchers so that culturally normal experiences and behaviours are not misconstrued as pathological.

First episode of psychosis

Clinical guidelines – access

- The community should be well informed

about psychotic disorders and how to obtain effective help. Community-wide initiatives to fight stigma associated with psychosis are required.
- Primary health care professionals should be competent in eliciting and recognizing the early clinical features of psychotic disorder, just as they are expected to detect new cases of potentially serious and life-threatening physical illnesses such as diabetes and hypertension.
- Enhanced undergraduate and postgraduate medical education and close links between primary and specialist mental health services are vital.
- Mental health services should provide user-friendly easy access to assessment and treatment for people who may be experiencing a first episode of psychosis. Assessment should be timely, depending on urgency, and flexible in terms of location.
- Ideally, treatment should commence prior to the development of a crisis such as self-harm, violence or aggression, substance misuse and its consequences, or vocational failure. Early intervention has the potential to allow engagement outside these emotionally-charged situations, providing a safer and more positive start to treatment. Inpatient care and tranquillizing medication are less likely to be needed if early intervention can be achieved.

- Families should be included in the assessment process and treatment plan, and this may be particularly relevant in developing countries.

Clinical guidelines – location of treatment

- Treatment should be provided in outpatient services or the home, if it is possible to give effective intervention in these settings, in order to minimize trauma, disruption and anxiety for the patient and the family.
- Inpatient care may be required if there is a significant risk of self-harm or aggression, if the level of support in the community is insufficient, or if the degree of crisis is too great for the family to manage. A psychosocial element to treatment is essential to manage the crises that face patients and families who are attempting to cope with a disturbing situation.
- Inpatient care should ideally be provided in units that provide services targeting early psychosis; the age and developmental stage of patients will also need to be taken into account.
- Inpatient units should be small in size and adequately staffed so that nursing of highly distressed or agitated young people is possible without locking the unit. A secure area is necessary so that care can be provided for aggressive or manic patients without harming or disturbing other patients.
- When it is not possible to offer an inpatient care in an early psychosis unit, a special section may be created in a general acute unit for young recent-onset patients. In addition to the practical and social effects, this symbolically communicates that young people differ in both needs and prognosis from older patients with chronic conditions.
- Some settings provide acute day services and, if specialized early psychosis care is available, may be an appropriate alternative to inpatient admission.
- If attempts to engage the person in treatment fail and the person remains actively psychotic, in most cases the person has a right to be treated on an involuntary basis (depending on local mental health legislation).

Clinical guidelines – initial management

- Before initiating treatment, it is important to consider physical illnesses that can cause psychosis.
- Extrapyramidal side effects from antipsychotic treatment should be avoided in order to encourage future adherence to medication. Although typical antipsychotics may be as efficacious as atypical antipsychotics in reducing positive

psychotic symptoms, they are frequently less well tolerated even at low doses. For this reason alone, atypical antipsychotics should be used as first-line therapy, commencing with a low dose and titrating upwards very slowly over a period of several weeks ('start low, go slow').

- Examples of appropriate initial target doses for most patients are risperidone 2 mg/day or olanzapine 7.5–10.0 mg/day. Initial target doses of other medications such as quetiapine, ziprasidone and amisulpride are yet to be established. Half to two-thirds of patients might be expected to achieve a good response in positive psychotic symptoms within 3 weeks at the initial dose, but if necessary the doses can be increased to 4 mg/day risperidone or 20 mg/day olanzapine. The level of clinical response and risk should be assessed frequently, but the dose of the antipsychotic should be increased only at widely spaced intervals (after initial titration, usually 14–21 days) if the response has been inadequate, and then only within the limits of sedation and the emergence of extrapyramidal side effects. However, extrapyramidal side effects should not be tolerated. If the response is not adequate at therapeutic doses by 6–8 weeks, another atypical antipsychotic should be tried. When use of typical antipsychotics is unavoidable, they should be commenced at very low doses (1–2 mg haloperidol or equivalent) and titrated very slowly within the limits of extrapyramidal side effects. Generally this will be a maximum of 4–6 mg haloperidol or equivalent in first-episode psychosis.

- Low doses of antipsychotic medication will not have a rapid effect on distress, insomnia and behavioural disturbances secondary to psychosis; skilled nursing care, a safe and supportive environment, and regular and liberal doses of benzodiazepines are essential interim components of management in many cases. Although some atypical antipsychotics have initial sedative side effects, treatment of psychosis should be separated conceptually from the need for tranquillization.

- If positive psychotic symptoms persist after a trial of two first-line atypical antipsychotics (around 12 weeks), the reasons for the failure of treatment should be reviewed. Possible contributing factors include adherence problems, family stresses and substance misuse. Slow recovery or early treatment resistance of this kind is of concern and requires more intensive intervention. Clozapine and cognitive–behavioural therapy for persistent symptoms are obvious alternatives to consider.

- Supportive crisis intervention, psychoeducation and cognitive therapy should be offered from early in the acute phase to facilitate recovery and acceptance of treatment. Specific psychosocial strategies should be employed when poor compliance, family stresses, increased suicide risk and substance misuse occur.

- Families are usually in crisis at the point of initiation of treatment and require emotional support and practical advice.

- Families and other members of the person's social network, possibly including friends, teachers and employers, should be progressively informed and educated about the nature of the problem, treatments and the outcomes expected.

- If there are frequent relapses or slow recovery, a more intensive and prolonged psychoeducational and supportive intervention for families may be required. A calm and optimistic approach is vital, especially if the early course is stormy or there are additional family problems or secondary consequences of untreated psychosis.

- Family therapy may be indicated when there is a high degree of distress in the family.

- Structured group programmes tailored to the immediate needs of the patient should be available.

Recovery (6–18 months) and the critical period (up to 5 years)

The time periods of 6–18 months for 'recovery' and up to 5 years as the 'critical period' are speculative. Time for remission of symptoms and risk of recurrence is highly variable and largely unknown.

Background

- It is essential that high-quality and intensive biopsychosocial care is provided continuously and assertively during the critical years after the onset psychosis. This standard is rarely met, because patients are usually required to manifest negative sequelae such as relapse, suicide attempts or severe disability before care is provided in a reactive and 'too little, too late' manner.

- Attempts should be made to ensure continuity of care, with 'treating clinicians' remaining constant for at least the first 18 months of treatment.

- Relapses are common during the first few years after the onset of a psychotic disorder and the vulnerability to relapse persists in about 80% of patients.

- Consumers and families must be involved and empowered.

Clinical guidelines

- The impact of the prodromal phase and the psychosis itself on the person, on the family, and on developmental and vocational tasks should be determined. Strategies offered within a case management model may include supportive psychotherapy, with an active problem-solving orientation, and negotiating occupational pursuits, including employment and/or education.
- Families should be provided with ongoing support and information, wherever possible in a partnership that involves the patient, family members and treating clinicians.
- Severe and potentially recurrent and disabling disorders of any kind in an adolescent or young adult can destabilize and distort the complex and often strained process of separation and individuation from the family. It is important to work within this context and not to misinterpret genuine attempts to cope.
- Psychological and psychosocial treatments should be core elements in the critical period and should be used to assist resolution of enduring positive and negative symptoms, the management of secondary comorbidity, and the promotion of recovery and positive mental health. Recovery work should emphasize the need to find meaning and develop mastery in relation to the psychotic experience.

- Multi-family groups (with or without the patient present) which have a psychoeducation focus should be provided.
- Depression, suicide risk, substance misuse and social anxiety in the patient should be identified and actively treated.
- Side effects of antipsychotic medication such as weight gain, sexual dysfunction and sedation can retard recovery and should be monitored regularly. Once psychosis has achieved a sustained remission, slow reduction of antipsychotic medication should be tried, with the aim of determining the minimal dose required.
- A balance is needed between vigilance for early signs of relapse and 'space' to recover and resume the challenges of normal development.
- Antipsychotic medication reduces the risk of relapse in the early years after onset and, particularly when there is a diagnosis of schizophrenia, should be considered as an essential basis for sustained recovery. Relapse is distressing and may increase the risk of treatment resistance and other 'collateral damage', including worsening stigma.
- The optimal length of time that maintenance antipsychotic treatment is needed to minimize risk of relapse in first episode psychosis is not known. Strong recommendations cannot be made about the optimal duration of maintenance treatment, although current clinical

practice varies from recommending continuation for 1 year after treatment initiation to indefinite duration of antipsychotic maintenance treatment. Against advice many young patients wish to cease medication. Individuals who elect to cease medication (prematurely or otherwise) should continue to be monitored frequently and receive ongoing support. In all instances, careful psychoeducation about the risks and possible manifestations of relapse should be provided, accompanied by frequent review and support with unhindered access to early psychiatric treatment in the event of relapse.

- In the absence of clear evidence about when to cease antipsychotic medication it is pragmatic to take into account the severity of the first episode. For example, a fully remitted patient may be presented the option of gradually withdrawing medication after full remission for 12 months; if the first psychotic episode was severe and slow to respond, continuation of medication for a 2-year period following remission might be suggested. If the patient makes an incomplete recovery but has benefited significantly from medication, then it should be continued for at least 2–5 years. Long-term medication is advisable for individuals who experience frequent relapses.
- Early warning signs of relapse should be discussed with the patient and family.

- If a patient who rejects treatment has persistent symptoms or experiences frequent relapses, with a pattern of high-risk, suicidal or aggressive behaviour, and is poorly engaged in treatment, then involuntary community treatment with or without depot medication may be required. This undesirable outcome should be considered to be time limited to allow intervention and/or time to assist with acceptance of treatment recommendations. Involuntary and other restrictive treatment practices should be subject to frequent review and a planned termination date.
- Patients should remain in comprehensive, multidisciplinary, specialist mental health care throughout the early years of psychosis and, once their acute symptoms improve, not be discharged or transferred to primary care without continuing specialist involvement. However, partnerships can be established between a specialist centre, primary care and other agencies that can contribute to optimal care. First-episode psychosis is difficult to treat well, confers high levels of risk, and is the phase with the potential for greatest cost-effectiveness of treatment. To treat in a reactive manner is less effective and misses the best opportunity for enhancing outcomes and quality of life for patients and families.
- For a subgroup of patients (e.g. patients with personality issues and/or enduring

positive symptoms) long-term psychotherapy may be indicated.

- Good relations between specialist early intervention services and general psychiatric services need to be fostered in order to facilitate the eventual transfer of care for a significant subgroup of individuals, because early intervention services are, by definition, time limited.

- Consumers and families with recent experience of early psychosis should be encouraged to participate in the development and monitoring of early psychosis services.

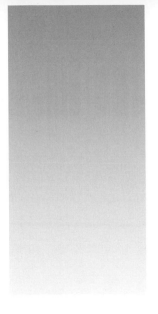

Appendix 1 – Psychoeducation resource material for early psychosis – source details

Something is Not Quite Right – pamphlet advising on when and how to get help if psychiatric illness is suspected. Published by: SANE Australia, P.O. Box 226, South Melbourne 3205, Victoria, Australia.
Tel: (03) 9682 5933, Fax: (03) 9682 5944.
www.sane.org

A Stitch in Time: Psychosis . . . Get Help Early – information kit (series of three videos and a booklet for general practitioners).
The aim of this kit is to raise awareness and provide information about psychosis and the importance of early detection and intervention. The material in the kit is available individually or as a complete package.
Published by: EPPIC for Psychiatric Services Branch, Victorian Government Department of Health and Community Services, September 1994.
Order form available from: EPPIC Statewide Services, Locked Bag 10, Parkville, Victoria, Australia 3052.
Tel: (03) 9342 2832, Fax: (03) 9342 2941.
www.eppic.org.au

A Stitch in Time: Psychosis . . . Get Help Early –
information sheets:
No. 1: *What is Psychosis?*
No. 2: *Recovering from Psychosis*
No. 3: *Getting Help Early*
No. 4: *How Can I Help Someone With Psychosis?*
Download from www.eppic.org.au
Bulk orders available via EPPIC (contact details – page 157).

SANE Australia (2000). The SANE Guide to Psychosis
Published by: SANE Australia (contact details – page 157).

Mood Swings and Mental Health: Information for Sufferers and Carers – Hovel J, Player J, eds
(ISBN 0 646 064037). Published by ARAFEMI, 1991.
Contact: ARAFEMI Victoria, Suite 1, 1091 Toorak Road, Camberwell 3124, Victoria, Australia.
Tel: (03) 9889 3733, Fax (03) 9889 2878.
www.vicnet.net.au/~arafemi

The Alice Guide to Psychosis (1996) – software and booklet
Available from: SANE Australia (contact details – page 157).

Cannabis and Psychosis Fact Sheet and *Booklet*
Download from
http://www.dhs.vic.gov.au/phd/hdev/cannabis

Trips and Journeys: Personal Accounts of Early Psychosis (2000) (EPPIC 2000a)
Order form available from: EPPIC (contact details – page 157).

Holding On to What is Real: A Video about Schizophrenia
Available from: Marcom Projects, P.O. Box 4215, Loganholme 4129, Queensland, Australia.
Tel: (07) 3801 5600, Fax: (07) 3801 5622.
www.marcom.com.au

Psychosis and Schizophrenia – Watkins J, 1999
(ISBN 0 646 118757). Published by and available from: Schizophrenia Fellowship of Victoria Inc.
www.sfv.org.au

Living with Schizophrenia: A Holistic Approach to Understanding, Preventing and Recovering from Negative Symptoms – Watkins J, 1996
(ISBN 0 85572 272X).
Published by: Hill of Content Publishing Company Pty Ltd, 86 Bourke Street, Melbourne, Australia.
Tel: (03) 9662 9472, Fax (03) 96622527.
e-mail: hoc@collinsbooks.com.au

Appendix 2 – Summary of recommendations from Australian Clinical Guidelines for Early Psychosis

Key elements of best practice for first onset psychosis

The National Clinical Guidelines for First Onset Psychosis outline 10 clinical practice guidelines for use by mental health professionals.

- Identifying, monitoring and providing needs-based care during a potential prodromal phase in early psychosis are optimal. Intervention during the prodromal phase may help to prevent the onset of psychosis.
- Mental Health Services are accessible and provide a timely assessment for people experiencing, or significantly at risk of, their first episode of psychosis and their families. Reducing delays into treatment through a clearly defined process of entry into specialist services can have positive outcomes, such as reducing the risk of relapse.
- Consumers and their carers receive a comprehensive, timely and accurate assessment and a regular review of progress. Assessment procedures for clients experiencing first onset psychosis should incorporate strategies to promote engagement.

- A case manager/mental health practitioner and treating psychiatrist should be allocated to each client upon entry to the service and provide a range of services to meet the needs of the client and their family and carers. The overarching goal of the case manager is the promotion of recovery and prevention of relapse and ongoing disability.
- Psychopharmacological interventions are to be provided during the acute phase and ongoing management of recovery for psychosis. The aim of psychopharmacology in first onset psychosis should be to maximise the therapeutic benefit for the client while minimising the side effects.
- Psychological interventions are provided as part of the acute and ongoing management of recovery from psychosis. The benefits of using psychological approaches to promote recovery are emerging.
- Family and carers are involved in the assessment, treatment and recovery process in episodes of acute psychosis. Families and carers play a vital role in supporting the client and facilitating engagement in treatment and thereby minimising long-term morbidity.
- Psychoeducation for clients and families is an essential component of the treatment process in early psychosis. Psychoeducation aims to develop a shared

and increased understanding of the illness for both the client and their family.
- A comprehensive range of group programs specifically tailored to the needs of people with early psychosis should be available. Group work interventions for people experiencing early psychosis can be both efficient and effective in promoting recovery and involvement in community life, reducing the development of disability and facilitating the achievement of personal goals and vocational goals.
- Clients should receive treatment in the least restrictive manner wherever possible. Choice of treatment setting is a very important component in the overall management of people with first onset psychosis. While the decision regarding treatment setting should be based on the level of severity of presentation, and the assessed level of risk, the optimal treatment setting is considered to be the client's home.

From: New South Wales Health Department (2000b). Getting in Early: A Framework for Early Intervention and Prevention in Mental Health for Young People in New South Wales (NSW Health Department, Sydney, Australia (www.hprb.health.nsw.gov.au/public-health). Reproduced with permission of the Centre for Mental Health, NSW Health Department.

Appendix 3 – Euro FESN Consensus: Optimum First Episode Care

1. Detection
   - public awareness
   - strategy for high risk cases
   - family practitioner training
   - swift response of acceptable assessment team

2. Acute management
   - appropriate assessments, including DUP
   - effective and acceptable drug treatment
   - effective psychological intervention
   - family support and psychoeducation
   - community treatment prioritised

3. Managing complications
   - monitor and address depressive symptoms
   - early use of clozapine for persisting symptoms
   - access to dual diagnosis services
   - compliance therapy
   - CBT for persisting symptoms

4. Sustaining remission
   - acceptable drug maintenance

- early signs monitoring
- family support
- continued psychosocial and psychological intervention

Reproduced with permission of S Lewis, from: *First in Line*, February 2000 (Euro FESN newsletter).

References

Addington J, Addington D (2001a) Early intervention for psychosis: The Calgary Early Psychosis Treatment and Prevention Program. *Canadian Psychiatric Association Bulletin* 33:11–16.

Addington J, Addington D (2001b) Impact of an early psychosis program on substance use. *Psychiatr Rehabil J*; 25:60–67.

Addington J, Jones B, Ko T, Addington D (in press) Family intervention in an early psychosis program. *Psychiatric Rehabil Skills*.

Aitchison KJ, Meehan K, Murray RM (1999) *First Episode Psychosis.* London: Martin Dunitz.

Alanen YO, Ugelstad E, Armelius BA et al (1994) Early treatment for schizophrenic patients: Scandinavian psychotherapeutic approaches. Oslo: Scandinavian University Press.

Albiston DJ, Francey SM, Harrigan SM (1998) Group programmes for recovery from early psychosis. *Br J Psychiatry* 172 (suppl 33):117–121.

American Psychiatric Association (1987) DSM-III-R: Diagnostic and Statistical Manual of Mental Disorders (3rd ed, revised). Washington, DC: American Psychiatric Publishing, Inc.

Amminger GP, Harris M, Elkins K et al. Treated incidence of first-episode psychosis in the catchment area of EPPIC, 1997–2000: an analysis of age- and sex-rates. Manuscript submitted for publication.

Andrews G, Peters L, Teesson M (1995) *Measurement of Consumer Outcome in Mental Health.* Canberra: Australian Government Publishing Service.

Australian Bureau of Statistics (2000) *Population by Age and Sex (30 June 1999; catalogue number 3235.2)*. Canberra: Commonwealth Government of Australia. (ISSN 1329–4105.)

Bell RQ (1992) Multiple-risk cohorts and segmenting risk as solutions to the problem of false positives in risk for the major psychoses. *Psychiatry* 55:370–381.

Bermanzohn PC, Porto L, Siris SG et al (2001) Hierarchy, reductionism and 'comorbidity' in the diagnosis of schizophrenia. In: Hwang MY, Bermanzohn PC, eds, *Management of Schizophrenia with Comorbid Conditions*. Washington, DC: American Psychiatric Publishing, Inc.

Birchwood M (1999) Early intervention in psychosis: the critical period. In: McGorry PD, Jackson HJ, eds, *Recognition and Management of Early Psychosis: A Preventive Approach*. New York: Cambridge University Press; 226–264.

Birchwood M (2000) The critical period for early intervention in psychosis. In: Birchwood M, Fowler D, Jackson C, eds, *Early Intervention in Psychosis: A Guide to Concepts Evidence And Intervention*. Chichester: Wiley; 28–63.

Birchwood M, Macmillan F (1993) Early intervention in schizophrenia. *Aust NZ J Psychiatry* 27:374–378.

Birchwood M, McGorry P, Jackson H (1997) Early intervention in schizophrenia [editorial]. *Br J Psychiatry* 170:2–5.

Birchwood M, Todd P, Jackson C (1998) Early intervention in psychosis: the critical period hypothesis. *Br J Psychiatry* 172(Suppl 33):53–59.

Birchwood M, Fowler D, Jackson C, eds (2000) *Early Intervention in Psychosis: A Guide to Concepts Evidence And Intervention*. Chichester: Wiley.

Brunner R, Parzer P, Mundt C, Resch F (1998) Psychotherapeutische aspekte in der stationären behandlung akutpsychiatrisch erkrankter jugendlicher. *Psychiatr Prax* 25:274–278.

Burgess P, Pirkis J (1999) The currency of case management: benefits and costs. *Curr Opin Psychiatry* 12:195–199.

Cameron DE (1938) Early schizophrenia. *Am J Psychiatry* 95:567–578.

Carbone S, Harrigan S, McGorry PD et al (1999) Duration of untreated psychosis and 12-month outcome in first-episode psychosis: the impact of treatment approach. *Acta Psychiatr Scand* 100:96–104.

Carr JV, Donovan P (1992) Psychiatry in general practice. A pilot scheme using the liaison attachment model. *Med J Aust* 156:379–382.

Carr V, Halpin S, Lau N et al (2000) A risk factor screening and assessment protocol for schizophrenia and related psychosis. *Aust NZ J Psychiatry* 34(Suppl.):170–180.

Catts SV, O'Donnell M, Spencer EA, Stewart KD (in press) Early psychosis intervention in routine service environments: implications for case management and routine service evaluation. In: Kashima H, Falloon IRH, Mizuno M, Asai M, eds, *Comprehensive Treatment of Schizophrenia: Keio University Symposia for Life Sciences and Medicine*, vol 8. Tokyo: Springer Verlag.

Chen EYH (1998) Early intervention in schizophrenia: rationale and practice. *Hong Kong Med J* 5:57–62.

Chen EYH, Dunn ELW, Chen RYL et al (1999) Duration of untreated psychosis and symptomatic outcome amongst first episode schizophrenic patients in Hong Kong. *Schizophr Res* 36:15.

Copolov DL, McGorry PD, Keks N et al (1989) Origins and establishment of the schizophrenia research programme at Royal Park Psychiatric Hospital. *Aust NZ J Psychiatry* 23:443–451.

Craig TJ, Bromet EJ, Fennig S et al (2000) Is there an association between duration of untreated psychosis and 24-month clinical outcome in a first-admission series? *Am J Psychiatry* 157:60–66.

Cullberg J, Thorén G, Åbb S, Svedberg B (2000) Integrating intensive psychosocial and low-dose neuroleptic treatment: a three-year follow-up. In: Martindale B, Bateman A, Crowe M, Margison F, eds, *Psychosis: Psychological Approaches and their Effectiveness.* London: Gaskell; 200–209.

Cullberg J, Levander S, Holmqvist R et al (in press) *Crisis intervention, small residential home, and low dose antipsychotic medication for a total population of first episode psychosis patients: one year results from the Parachute project and a comparison group.*

Dawson S (1997) Inhabiting different worlds: how can research relate to practice [editorial]. *Qual Health Care* 6:177–178.

De Hert M, Magiels G, Thys E (2000) *The Secret of the Brain Chip.* Antwerp, Belgium: EPO publishing.

Drake RE, Gates C, Cotton PG, Whitaker A (1984) Suicide among schizophrenics: who is at risk? *J Nerv Ment Dis* 172:613–617.

Driessen G, Gunther N, Bak M et al (1998) Characteristics of early- and late-diagnosed schizophrenia: implications for first-episode studies. *Schizophr Res* 33:27–34.

Drury V (2000) Cognitive behaviour therapy in early psychosis. In: Birchwood M, Fowler D, Jackson C, eds, *Early Intervention in Psychosis: A Guide to Concepts, Evidence and Intervention.* Chichester: Wiley; 185–212.

Drury V, Birchwood M, Cochrane R, Macmillan F (1996a) Cognitive therapy and recovery from acute psychosis: a controlled trial. I: Impact on psychotic symptoms. *Br J Psychiatry* 169:593–601.

Drury V, Birchwood M, Cochrane R, Macmillan F (1996b) Cognitive therapy and recovery from acute psychosis: a controlled trial. II: Impact on recovery time. *Br J Psychiatry* 169:602–607.

Eaton WW (1999) Evidence for universality and uniformity of schizophrenia around the world: assessment and implications. In: Gattaz WF, Hafner H, eds, *Search for the Causes of*

Schizophrenia. Darmstadt, Steinkopff (Springer Verlag) 21–33.

Eaton WW, Badawi M, Melton B (1995) Prodromes and precursors: epidemiologic data for primary prevention of disorders with slow onset. *Am J Psychiatry* 152:967–972.

Edwards J, Harris M, Herman A (in press a) The early psychosis prevention and intervention centre. In: Ogura C, ed, *Recent Advances in Early Intervention and Prevention in Psychiatric Disorders* Tokyo: Seiwa Shoten Publishers Tokyo.

Edwards J, McGorry PD (1998) Early intervention in psychotic disorders: a critical step in the prevention of psychological morbidity In: Perris C, McGorry PD, eds, *Cognitive Psychotherapy of Psychotic and Personality Disorders.* Chichester: Wiley; 167–195.

Edwards J, Francey SM, McGorry PD, Jackson HJ (1994) Early psychosis prevention and intervention: evolution of a comprehensive community-based specialised service. *Behav Change* 11:223–233.

Edwards J, Maude D, McGorry PD et al (1998) Prolonged recovery in first-episode psychosis. *Br J Psychiatry* 172(suppl):107–116.

Edwards J, Cocks J, Bott J (1999) Preventive case management in first-episode psychosis. In: McGorry PD, Jackson HJ, eds, *Recognition and Management of Early Psychosis: A Preventive Approach.* New York: Cambridge University Press; 308–337.

Edwards J, McGorry PD, Pennell K (2000) Models of early intervention in psychosis: an analysis of service approaches. In: Birchwood M, Fowler D, Jackson C, eds, *Early Intervention in Psychosis: A Guide to Concepts Evidence and Intervention.* Chichester: Wiley; 281–314.

Edwards J, Hinton M, Elkins K, Athanasopoulos O (in press b) Cannabis and first-episode psychosis: The CAP project. In: Graham H, Mueser K, Birchwood M, Copello A, eds, *Substance Misuse in*

Psychosis: Approaches to Treatment and Service Delivery. Chichester: Wiley.

Edwards J, Maude D, Herrmann-Doig T et al (in press c) A service response to prolonged recovery in early psychosis. *Psychiatr Serv.*

EPPIC (1994) *A Stitch in Time: Psychosis . . . Get Help Early: A Booklet for General Practitoners.* Melbourne: Early Psychosis Prevention and Intervention Centre.

EPPIC (1997a) *Psychoeducation in Early Psychosis: Manual 1 in a Series of Early Psychosis Manuals.* Melbourne: Early Psychosis Prevention and Intervention Centre, Statewide Services.

EPPIC (1997b) *Working with Families in Early Psychosis: Manual 2 in a Series of Early Psychosis Manuals.* Melbourne: Early Psychosis Prevention and Intervention Centre, Statewide Services.

EPPIC (2000a) *Trips and Journeys – Personal Accounts of Early Psychosis.* Melbourne: Early Psychosis Prevention and Intervention Centre.

EPPIC (2000b) *Working with Groups in Early Psychosis: Manual 3 in a Series of Early Psychosis Manuals.* Melbourne: Early Psychosis Prevention and Intervention Centre.

EPPIC (2001a) *Case Management in Early Psychosis: A Handbook.* Melbourne: Early Psychosis Prevention and Intervention Centre.

EPPIC (2001b) *Youth Pack.* Melbourne: Early Psychosis Prevention and Intervention Centre.

EPPIC (2002a) *Cognitively-Oriented Psychotherapy for Early Psychosis: Manual 4 in a Series of Early Psychosis Manuals.* Melbourne: Early Psychosis Prevention and Intervention Centre.

EPPIC (2002b) *Cannabis and Psychosis: An Early Psychosis Treatment Manual and Video.* Melbourne: Early Psychosis Prevention and Intervention Centre.

EPPIC (2002c) *Prolonged Recovery in Early Psychosis: A Treatment Manual and Video.*

Melbourne: Early Psychosis Prevention and Intervention Centre.

EPPIC (2002d) *Suicide Prevention in Young People with a Mental Illness: A Clinician's Guide.* Melbourne: Early Psychosis Prevention and Intervention Centre.

Epstein I (in press) Using available clinical information in a practice-based research: mining for silver while dreaming for gold. In: Epstein I, Blumenfield S, eds, *Clinical Data-Mining in Practice-Based Research: Social Work in Hospital Settings.* Binghampton, NY: Haworth Press.

Falloon IRH (1992) Early intervention for first episodes of schizophrenia: a preliminary exploration. *Psychiatry* 55:4–15.

Falloon IRH, Kydd RR, Coverdale JH, Laidlaw TM (1996) Early detection and intervention for initial episodes of schizophrenia. *Schizophr Bull* 22:271–282.

Falloon IRH, Coverdale JH, Laidlaw TM et al (1998) Early intervention for schizophrenic disorders: implementing optimal strategies in routine clinical services. *Br J Psychiatry* 172 (suppl):33–38.

Fennig S, Kovasznay B, Rich C et al (1994) Six-month stability of psychiatric diagnoses in first-admission patients with psychosis. *Am J Psychiatry* 151:1200–1208.

Fenton WS (1997) Course and outcome in schizophrenia. *Curr Opin Psychiatry* 10:40–44.

Fenton WS (2000) Evolving perspectives on individual psychotherapy for schizophrenia. *Schizophr Bull* 26:137–139.

Fitzgerald P, Kulkarni J (1998) Home-oriented management programme for people with early psychosis. *Br J Psychiatry* 172 (suppl):39–44.

Frances A (1998) Problems in defining clinical significance in epidemiological studies. *Arch Gen Psychiatry* 55:119.

Garety P, Jolley S (2000) Early intervention in psychosis [editorial]. *Psychiatr Bull* 24:321–323.

Garety PA, Fowler D, Kuipers E (2000). Cognitive–behavioural therapy for people with psychosis. In: Martindale D, Bateman A, Crowe M, Margison F, eds, *Psychosis: Psychological Approaches and their Effectiveness.* London: Gaskell; 30–49.

Gitlin M, Nuechterlein K, Subotnik KL et al (2001). Clinical outcome following neuroleptic discontinuation in patients with remitted recent – onset schizophrenia. *Am J Psychiatry,* **158**: 1835–1842.

Gleeson J, Jackson HJ, Stavely H, Burnett P (1999) Family intervention in early psychosis. In: McGorry PD, Jackson HJ, eds, *Recognition and Management of Early Psychosis: A Preventive Approach.* New York: Cambridge University Press; 376–406.

Green LW, Kreuter MW (1999). *Health Promotion Planning: An Educational and Ecological Approach,* 3rd edn. Mountain View: Mayfield Publishing Company.

Grimshaw JM, Hutchinson A (1995) Clinical practice guidelines – do they enhance value for money in health care? *Br Med Bull* 51:927–940.

Haddock G, Morrison AP, Hopkins R et al (1988). Individual cognitive–behavioural interventions in early psychosis. *Br J Psychiatry* 172 (suppl): 93–100.

Häfner H, Riecher-Rössler A, Hambrecht M et al (1992) IRAOS: An instrument for the assessment of onset and early course of schizophrenia. *Schizophr Res* 6:209–223.

Häfner H, Nowotny B, Löffler W et al (1995) When and how does schizophrenia produce social deficits? *Eur Arch Psychiatry Clin Neurosci* 246: 17–28.

Häfner H, Löffler W, Maurer K et al (1999) Depression, negative symptoms, social stagnation and social decline in the early course of schizophrenia. *Acta Psychiatr Scand* 100:105–118.

Hambrecht M, Häfner H (1996) Substance abuse and the onset of schizophrenia. *Biol Psychiatry* 40: 1155–1163.

Hamilton Wilson J, Hobbs H (1995) Therapeutic partnership: a model for clinical practice. *J Psychosoc Nurs* 33:27–30.

Hamilton Wilson J, Hobbs H (1999) The family educator: a professional resource for families. *J Psychosoc Nurs* 37:22–27.

Harvey HD, Keefe RSE (2001) Studies of cognitive change in patients with schizophrenia following novel antipsychotic treatment. *Am J Psychiatry* 158:176–184.

Hegarty J, Baldessarini R, Tohen M et al (1994) One hundred years of schizophrenia: a meta-analysis of the outcome literature. *Am J Psychiatry* 151:1409–1416.

Helgason L (1990) Twenty years follow-up of first psychiatric presentation for schizophrenia: what could have been prevented? *Acta Psychiatr Scand* 81: 231–235.

Herrmann-Doig TL, Maude D, Edwards J (2001) *Systematic Treatment of Persistent Psychosis (STOPP): A Psychological Approach to Facilitating Recovery in First-Episode Psychosis.* In press.

Ho B-C, Andreasen NC, Flaum M et al (2000). Untreated initial psychosis: Its relation to quality of life and symptom remission in first episode schizophrenia. *Am J Psychiatry,* 157:808–815.

Hobbs H, Hamilton Wilson J, Archie S (1999) The Alumni Program: redefining continuity of care in psychiatry. *J Psychosoc Nurs* 37:23–29.

Hodges CA, Sanci LA, McGorry PD (1999) Adolescent mental health: early intervention in primary care. *Mod Med Aust* Oct:74–83.

Hogarty GE, Anderson CM, Reiss DJ et al (1986) Family psychoeducation, social skills training, and maintenance chemotherapy in the aftercare treatment of schizophrenia. 1. One-year effects of a controlled study on relapse and expressed emotion. *Arch Gen Psychiatry* **43**:633–642.

Howe D, Temple L, Mackso C, Teeson M (1999). *"Catch Us If U Can": Young People and Psychiatric Illness – Intervention and Assessment.* Gosford, NSW: Central Coast Health Service.

Hulbert CA, Jackson HJ, McGorry PD (1996) The relationship between personality and course and outcome in early psychosis: a review of the literature. *Clin Psychol Rev* **16**:707–727.

Ioannides T (Producer), Hexter I (Director) (1994a) *A Stitch in Time: Psychosis . . . Get Help Early: A Community Video.* Melbourne: Early Psychosis Prevention and Intervention Centre.

Ioannides T (Producer), Hexter I (Director) (1994b) *A Stitch in Time: Psychosis . . . Get Help Early: A Video About EPPIC.* Melbourne: Early Psychosis Prevention and Intervention Centre.

Ioannides T (Producer), Hexter I (Director) (1994c) *A Stitch in Time: Psychosis . . . Get Help Early: A Video for General Practitioners.* Melbourne: Early Psychosis Prevention and Intervention Centre.

Jablensky A (1997) The 100-year epidemiology of schizophrenia. *Schizophr Res* **28**:111–125.

Jablensky A, Sartorius N, Ernberg G et al (1992) Schizophrenia: manifestations incidence and course in different cultures. A World Health Organization 10-country study. *Psychol Med Monogr,* **190**:20–97.

Jablensky A, McGrath J, Herrman H et al (1999) *People Living with Psychotic Illness: An Australian Study 1997–98.* Canberra: Department of Health and Aged Care, Commonwealth of Australia.

Jackson C, Farmer A (1998) Early intervention in psychosis. *J Mental Health* **7**:157–164.

Jackson HJ, McGorry PD, Dudgeon P (1995) Prodromal symptoms of schizophrenia in first-episode patients: prevalence and specificity. *Compr Psychiatr* **36**:241–250.

Jackson H J, McGorry PD, Edwards J, Hulbert C (1996) Cognitively-oriented psychotherapy for early psychosis (COPE). In: Cotton P, Jackson J, eds, *Early Intervention and Preventative Application of Clinical Psychology.* Melbourne: Australian Psychological Society; 131–154.

Jackson HJ, McGorry PD, Edwards J et al (1998) Cognitively orientated psychotherapy for early psychosis (COPE): preliminary results. *Br J Psychiatr* **172** (suppl):93–100.

Jackson HJ, Edwards J, McGorry PD, Hulbert C (1999) Recovery from psychosis: psychological interventions. In: McGorry PD, Jackson HJ, eds, *Recognition and Management of Early Psychosis: A Preventive Approach.* New York: Cambridge University Press; 213–235.

Jackson HJ, Hulbert CA, Henry LP (2000) The treatment of secondary morbidity in first-episode psychosis. In: Birchwood M, Fowler D, Jackson C, eds, *Early Intervention in Psychosis: A Guide to Concepts Evidence and Intervention.* Chichester: Wiley; 281–314.

Jackson HJ, McGorry PD, Edwards J (2001a) Cognitively oriented psychotherapy for early psychosis (COPE): theory, praxis, outcome and challenges. In: Corrigan P, Penn D, eds, *Social Cognition and Schizophrenia.* Washington, DC: APA Press; 249–284.

Jackson H, McGorry P, Henry L et al (2001b) Cognitively oriented psychotherapy for early psychosis (COPE): a 1-year follow-up. *Br J Clin Psychol* **40**:57–70.

Jarskog LF, Mattioli MA, Perkins DO, Lieberman JA (2000) First-episode psychosis in a managed care setting: clinical management and research. *Am J Psychiatry* **157**:878–884.

Johannessen JO (2001) Early recognition and intervention: the key to success in the treatment of schizophrenia? *Dis Manag Health Outcomes* **9**: 317–327.

Johannessen JO, Larsen TK, McGlashan T (1999). Duration of untreated psychosis: an important target for intervention in schizophrenia? *Nord J Psychiatry* 53:275–283.

Johannessen JO, Larsen TK, McGlashan T, Vaglum P (2000) Early identification in psychosis: the TIPS project a multi-centre study in Scandinavia. In: Martindale D, Bateman A, Crowe M, Margison F, eds, *Psychosis: Psychological Approaches and Their Effectiveness.* London: Gaskell; 210–234.

Johannessen JO, Larsen TK, Horneland M et al (2001) The TIPS Project. A systematized program to reduce duration of untreated psychosis in first episode psychosis. In: Miller T, McGlashan TH, Mednick SA et al, eds, *Early Intervention in Psychotic Disorders.* Dordrecht: Kluwer Academic Publishers. 151–166.

Johannessen JO, Larsen TK, Horneland M et al (in press b). Early detection strategies for untreated psychosis. *Schizophr Res.*

Johnson DAW (1996) Peer review of 'Cognitive therapy and recovery from acute psychosis'. *Br J Psychiatry* 169:608–609.

Johnstone EC, Crow TJ, Johnson AL, Macmillan JF (1986). The Northwick Park study of first episodes of schizophrenia: 1. Presentation of the illness and problems relating to admission. *Br J Psychiatry* 148:115–120.

Jones PB, Bebbington P, Foerster A et al (1993) Premorbid social underachievement in schizophrenia: results from the Camberwell Collaborative Psychosis Study. *Br J Psychiatry* 162:65–71.

Jørgensen P, Nordentoft M, Abel MB et al (2000) Early detection and assertive community treatment of young psychotics: the OPUS Study. Rationale and design of the trial. *Soc Psychiatry Psychiatr Epidemiol* 35:283–287.

Jorm A, Korten AE, Jacomb PA et al (1997) 'Mental health literacy': a survey of the public's ability to recognise mental disorders and their beliefs about the effectiveness of treatment. *Med J Aust* 166:182–186.

Joyce C, Hurworth R (1998) *Evaluation of the National Early Psychosis Project: Final Report.* Melbourne: Centre for Program Evaluation, University of Melbourne.

Kane JM, Marder SR (1993) Psychopharmacologic treatment of schizophrenia. *Schizophr Bull* 19:287–302.

Kapur S, Zipursky RB, Remington G (1999) Comparison and theoretical implications of 5-HT2 and D2 receptor occupancy of clozapine, risperidone and olanzapine in schizophrenia: clinical and theoretical implications. *Am J Psychiatry* 156:286–293.

Kessler RC, Foster CL, Saunders WB, Stang PE (1995) Social consequences of psychiatric disorders. I Educational attainment. *Am J Psychiatry* 152:1026–1032.

Klosterkötter J (1998) Von der krankheitsbekämpung zur krankheitsverhütung. *Fortschr Neurol Psychiat* 66:366–377.

Kovasznay B, Fleischer J, Tanenberg-Karant M et al (1997) Substance use disorder and the early course of illness in schizophrenia and affective psychosis. *Schizophr Bull* 23:195–201.

Kraeplin E (1896). Dementia praecox. Translated into English, 1987. In: *The Clinical Roots of the Schizophrenia Concept.* Cutting J and Shepherd M (eds). Cambridge: Cambridge University Press.

Krausz M, Muller-Thomsen T, Maasen C (1995) Suicide among schizophrenic adolescents in the long-term course of illness. *Psychopathology* 28:95–103.

Krstev H, McGorry PD, Harrigan SM, Carbone S (2001a) *Early intervention in first-episode psychosis: The impact of a community development campaign.* Manuscript submitted for publication.

Krstev H, McGorry PD, Harrigan S, Haines S (2001b) *Preliminary evaluation of an early psychosis project within a mainstream setting*, Manuscript submitted for publication.

Kulkarni J (1999) Home-based treatment of first-episode psychosis. In: McGorry PD, Jackson HJ, eds, *Recognition and Management of Early Psychosis: A Preventive Approach*. New York: Cambridge University Press; 206–225.

Kulkarni J, Power P (1999) Initial management of first-episode psychosis. In: McGorry PD, Jackson HJ, eds, *Recognition and Management of Early Psychosis: A Preventive Approach*. New York: Cambridge University Press; 184–205.

Kundera M (1996) *The Book of Laughter and Forgetting*. London: Faber and Faber.

Larsen TK, McGlashan TH, Moe LC (1996) First-episode schizophrenia: I. Early course parameters. *Schizophr Bull* 22:241–256.

Larsen TK, Johannessen JO, Opjordsmoen S (1998) First-episode schizophrenia with long duration of untreated psychosis. *Br J Psychiatry* 172 (suppl):45–52.

Larsen TK, Johannessen JO, McGlashan T et al (2000a) Can duration of untreated psychosis be reduced? In: Birchwood M, Fowler D, Jackson C, eds, *Early Intervention in Psychosis: A Guide to Concepts Evidence and Intervention*. Chichester: Wiley; 143–165.

Larsen TK, Moe LC, Vibe-Hansen L, Johannessen JO (2000b) Premorbid functioning versus duration of untreated psychosis in 1 year outcome in first-episode psychosis. *Schizophr Res* 45:1–9.

Larsen TK, Friis S, Haahr U et al (2001a) Early detection and intervention in first-episode schizophrenia: a critical review. *Acta Psychiatr Scand* 103:323–334.

Larsen TK, McGlashan TH, Johannessen JO et al (2001b). Shortened duration of untreated first episode of psychosis: Changes in patient characteristics at treatment. *Am J Psychiatry* 158:1917–1919.

Lehman AF, Steinwachs DM and the Co-Investigators of the PORT Project (1998) At issue: translating research into practice: the Schizophrenia Patient Outcomes Research Team (PORT) treatment recommendations. *Schizophr Bull* 24: 1–10.

Lewis S, Drake R (2001) Commentary, Spencer et al (2001). *Adv Psychiatr Treat* 7:140–142.

Lewis SW, Tarrier N, Haddock G et al (manuscript submitted for publication). A multicentre, randomized controlled trial of a cognitive behaviour therapy in early schizophrenia: acute phase analysis.

Lewis SW, Tarrier N, Haddock G et al (2001) A randomised controlled trial of cognitive behaviour therapy in early schizophrenia. *Schizophr Res* 49 (suppl):263–264.

Lieberman JA (1996) Atypical antipsychotic drugs as a first-line treatment of schizophrenia: a rationale and hypotheses. *J Clin Psychiatry* 57:68–71.

Lieberman JA, Fenton WS (2000) Delayed detection of psychosis: causes, consequences, and effects on public health. *Am J Psychiatry* 157: 1727–1730.

Lieberman JM, Jody D, Geisler S et al (1993) Time course and biological correlates of treatment response in first-episode schizophrenia. *Arch Gen Psychiatry* 50:369–376.

Lincoln CV, McGorry PD (1995) Who cares? Pathways to psychiatric care for young people experiencing a first episode of psychosis. *Psychiatr Serv* 46:1166–1171.

Lincoln CV, McGorry PD (1999) Pathways to care in early psychosis: Clinical and consumer perspectives. In: McGorry PD, Jackson HJ, eds, *The Recognition and Management of Early Psychosis: A Preventative Approach*. Cambridge: Cambridge University Press, pp. 51–79.

Lincoln CV, Harrigan S, McGorry P (1998)

Understanding the topogaphy of the early psychosis pathways. *Br J Psychiatry* **172**(suppl 33):21–25.

Linszen D, Dingemans PM, Lenior ME (1994) Cannabis abuse and the course of recent-onset schizophrenic disorders. *Arch Gen Psychiatry* **51**: 273–279.

Loebel AD, Lieberman JA, Alvir MJ et al (1992) Duration of psychosis and outcome in first-episode schizophrenia. *Am J Psychiatry* **149**:1183–1188.

Lukoff D, Neuchterlein KH, Ventura J (1986) Manual for the Expanded Brief Psychiatric Scale. *Schizophr Bull* **12**:594–602.

Macmillan F, Shiers D (2000) The IRIS programme. In: Birchwood M, Fowler D, Jackson C, eds, *Early Intervention in Psychosis: A Guide to Concepts, Evidence and Intervention.* Chichester: Wiley; 281–314.

Mahy G, Mallett R, Leff J, Bhugra D (1999) First-contact incidence rate of schizophrenia on Barbados. *Br J Psychiatry* **175**:28–33.

Malla AK, Norman RMG (1999) Facing the challenges of intervening early in psychosis. *Annals RCPSC* **32**:394–397.

Malla AK, Norman RMG, Voruganti LP (1999) Improving outcome in schizophrenia: the case for early intervention. *Can Med Assoc J* **160**:843–846.

Malla AK, Norman RMG, McLean TS, McIntosh E (2001a) Impact of phase-specific treatment of first episode of psychosis on Wisconsin Quality of Life Index (client version). *Acta Psychiatr Scand* **103**: 355–361.

Malla AK, Norman RM, Scholten DJ et al (2001b) A comparison of long-term outcome in first-episode schizophrenia following treatment with risperidone or a typical antipsychotic. *J Clin Psychiatry* **62**: 179–184.

Malla AK, Norman RMG, Manchanda R et al (in press). One year outcome in first episode psychosis: influence of DUP and other predictors. *Schizophr Res.*

Manji HK, Moore GJ, Chen G (2000) Lithium up-regulates the cytoprotective protein Bcl-2 in the CNS in vivo: a role for neurotrophic and neuroprotective effects in manic depressive illness. *J Clin Psychiatry* **61**:82–96.

May R (2000) Routes to recovery: the roots of a clinical psychologist. *Clin Psychol Forum* **146**:6–10.

McEvoy JP, Hogarty GE, Steingard S (1991) Optimal dose of neuroleptic in acute schizophrenia: a controlled study of the neuroleptic threshold and higher haloperidol dose. *Arch Gen Psychiatry* **48**: 739–745.

McFarlane WR (2000) Psychoeducational multi-family groups: adaptations and outcomes. In: Martindale D, Bateman A, Crowe M, Margison F, eds, *Psychosis: Psychological Approaches and Their Effectiveness.* London: Gaskell; 68–95.

McFarlane WR (2001) Family-based treatment of prodromal and first-episode psychosis. In: Miller T, McGlashan TH, Mednick SA et al, eds, *Early Intervention in Psychotic Disorders.* Dordrecht: Kluwer Academic Publishers. 197–230.

McGlashan T, ed (1996) Issue theme: early detection and intervention in schizophrenia. *Schizophr Bull* **22**:197–352.

McGlashan T (1999) Duration of untreated psychosis in first episode schizophrenia: marker or determinant of course? *Biol Psychiatry* **46**:899–907.

McGlashan TH, Miller TJ, Woods SW et al (2001) A scale for the assessment of prodromal symptoms and states. In: Miller T, McGlashan TH, Mednick SA et al, eds, *Early Intervention in Psychotic Disorders.* Dordrecht: Kluwer Academic Publishers. 135–149.

McGorry PD (1992) The concept of recovery and secondary prevention in psychotic disorders. *Aust NZ J Psychiatry* **26**:3–17.

McGorry P (1995a) A treatment-relevant classification of psychotic disorders. *Aust NZ J Psychiatry* **29**:555–558.

McGorry PD (1995b) Psycho-education in first-episode psychosis: a therapeutic process. *Psychiatry* 58:329–344.

McGorry P (1998) Preventive strategies in early psychosis: verging on reality. *Br J Psychiatry* 172 (suppl 33):1–2.

McGorry PD (2000) The scope for preventive strategies in early psychosis: logic evidence and momentum. In: Birchwood M, Fowler D, Jackson C, eds, *Early Intervention in Psychosis: A Guide to Concepts, Evidence and Intervention.* Chichester: Wiley; 3–27.

McGorry PD (2001) Secondary prevention of mental disorders. In: Thornicroft G, Szmukler G, eds, *Textbook of Community Psychiatry.* Oxford: Oxford University Press. 495–508.

McGorry PD (in press) The detection and optimal management of early psychosis. In: Murray R, Lieberman J, eds, *Comprehensive Care of Schizophrenia.* London: Martin Dunitz.

McGorry PD, Edwards J (1997) *Early Psychosis Training Pack.* Macclesfield, UK: Gardiner-Caldwell. Download via www.eppic.org.au or www.futur.com

McGorry PD, Jackson HJ, eds (1999) *Recognition and Management of Early Psychosis: A Preventive Approach.* New York: Cambridge University Press.

McGorry PD, Singh BS (1995) Schizophrenia: risk and possibility of prevention. In: Raphael B, Burrows GD, eds, *Handbook of Studies on Preventive Psychiatry.* New York: Elsevier; 491–514.

McGorry PD, Coplov DL, Singh BS (1990a) Royal Park Multidiagnostic Instrument for Psychosis: Part I Rationale and review. *Schizophr Bull* 16:501–515.

McGorry PD, Singh BS, Copolov DL et al (1990b) Royal Park Multidiagnostic Instrument for Psychosis: Part II Development, reliability, and validity. *Schizophr Bull* 16:517–536.

McGorry PD, Chanen A, McCarthy E et al (1991)

Post-traumatic stress disorder following recent-onset psychosis: an unrecognised post-psychotic syndrome. *J Nerv Ment Dis* 179:253–258.

McGorry PD, McFarlane C, Patton G et al (1995) The prevalence of prodromal features of schizophrenia in adolescence: a preliminary survey. *Acta Psychiatr Scand* 92:241–249.

McGorry PD, Edwards J, Mihalopoulos C et al (1996) EPPIC: An evolving system of early detection and optimal management. *Schizophr Bull* 22:305–326.

McGorry PD, Henry L, Maude D, Phillips L (1998) Preventively-orientated psychological interventions in early psychosis. In: Perris C, McGorry PD, eds, *Cognitive Psychotherapy of Psychotic and Personality Disorders.* Chichester: Wiley; 213–236.

McGorry PD, Edwards J, Pennell K (1999) Sharpening the focus: early intervention in the real world. In: McGorry PD, Jackson HJ, eds, *Recognition and Management of Early Psychosis: A Preventive Approach.* New York: Cambridge University Press; 441–475.

McGorry PD, Phillips LJ, Yung AR (2001a) Recognition and treatment of the pre-psychotic phase of psychotic disorders: frontier or fantasy? In: Miller T, McGlashan TH, Mednick SA et al, eds, *Early Intervention in Psychotic Disorders.* Dordrecht: Kluwer Academic Publishers. 101–122.

McGorry PD, Yung AR, Phillips LJ et al (in press) Can first episode psychosis be delayed or prevented? A randomized controlled trial of interventions during the prepsychotic phase of schizophrenia and related psychoses. *Arch Gen Psychiatry.*

McGorry PD, Yung AR, Phillips LJ (2001b) 'Closing in': What features predict the onset of first-episode psychosis within an ultra-high-risk group? In: Zirpursky RB, Schulz SC, eds, *The Early Stages* of Schizophrenia. Washington, DC: American Psychiatric Publishing, Inc. 3–31.

McGorry PD, Yung A, Phillips L (2001c) Ethics and early intervention in psychosis: keeping up the pace and staying in step. Schizophr Res 51:17–29.

McGuire W (1984) Public communication as a strategy for inducing health-promoting behavioural change. Prev Med 13:299–319.

Meares A (1959) The diagnosis of prepsychotic schizophrenia. Lancet i:55–59.

Mechanic D (1996) Emerging issues in international mental health services research. Psychiatr Serv 47:371–375.

Meltzer HY (1995). Clozapine: is another view valid? Am J Psychiatry 152:821–823.

Meltzer HY, Okayli G (1995) Reduction of suicidality during clozapine treatment of neuroleptic-resistant schizophrenia: impact on risk-benefit assessment. Am J Psychiatry 152:183–190.

Mental Health Division, Health Department of Western Australia (2000) Early Episode Psychosis – Information/Policy Paper. Mental Health Division, Health Department of Western Australia.

Mental Health Evaluation and Community Consultation Unit (Mheccu) (1999) Early Psychosis Identification and Intervention Initiative: Towards a Framework and Best Practice Approach in Regional Implementation. Vancouver: University of British Columbia.

Mihalopoulos C, McGorry PD, Carter RC (1999) Is phase-specific community-oriented treatment of early psychosis an economically viable method of improving outcome? Acta Psychiatr Scand 100: 47–55.

Miller TJ, McGlashan TH, Woods SW et al (1999) Symptom assessment in schizophrenic prodromal states. Psychiatr Q 70:273–287.

Mrazek PJ, Haggerty RJ, eds (1994) Reducing Risks

for Mental Disorders: Frontiers for Preventive Intervention Research. Washington, DC: National Academy Press.

Mueser KT, Bond GR, Drake RE, Resnick SG (1998) Models of community care for severe mental illness: a review of research on case management. Schizophr Bull 24:37–74.

National Early Psychosis Project (1998) Getting in Early: Sally's Story: A Video for Mental Health Professionals. NSW Health Department, Sydney.

National Early Psychosis Project Clinical Guidelines Working Party (1998) Australian Clinical Guidelines for Early Psychosis. Melbourne: University of Melbourne.

New South Wales Health Department (2000a) Early Psychosis Area Programs and Services NSW: NSW Resource Document. Sydney: NSW Health Department.

New South Wales Health Department (2000b) Getting in Early: A Framework for Early Intervention and Prevention in Mental Health for Young People in New South Wales. Sydney: NSW Health Department. www.health.nsw.gov.au

Nordentoft M, Jeppesen P, Abel M-B et al (in press) OPUS-study: Suicidal behaviour, suicidal ideation, and hopelessness among first-episode psychotic patients. A one-year follow up of a randomised controlled trial. Br J Psychiatry.

Norman RMG, Malla AK (1993) Stressful life events and schizophrenia II: conceptual and methodological issues. Br J Psychiatry 162:166–174.

Norman RMG, Malla AK (2001) Duration of untreated psychosis: a critical examination of the concept and its importance. Psychol Med 31: 381–400.

Nuechterlein KH, Dawson ME (1984) A heuristic vulnerability stress model of schizophrenic episodes. Schizophr Bull 10:300–312.

Nuechterlein KH, Dawson ME, Gitlin M et al

(1992) Developmental processes in schizophrenic disorders: longitudinal studies of vulnerability and stress. *Schizophr Bull* 18:387–425.

Nyberg S, Farde L, Halldin C et al (1995) D2 dopamine receptor occupancy during low-dose treatment with haloperidol decanoate. *Am J Psychiatry* 152:173–178.

Owen JM, Rogers (1999) *Program Evaluation: Forms and Approaches,* 2nd edn. St Leonards: Allen & Unwin.

Padmavathi R, Rajkumar S, Srinivasan T (1998) Schizophrenic patients who were never treated – a study in an Indian urban community. *Psychol Med* 28:1113–1117.

Parker G, Roy K, Hadzi-Pavlovic D, Pedic F (1992) Psychotic depression: a meta-analysis of physical treatments. *J Affect Disord* 24:17–24.

Pennell K, McGorry PD (2001) *Australian National Early Psychosis Project: Its Activities, Outcomes and Recommendations.* Melbourne: University of Melbourne.

PEPP (2000a) *Prevention and Early Intervention Program for Psychosis: Screening, Assessment and Treatment Manuals.* London, Ontario: London Health Sciences Centre.

PEPP (2000b) *Working Together: Things Can Get Better. A Program for Families Dealing with Early Psychosis.* London, Ontario: London Health Sciences Centre.

Phillips LJ, Yung AR, McGorry PD (2000) Identification of young people at risk of psychosis: validation of Personal Assessment and Crisis Evaluation Clinic intake criteria. *Aust NZ J Psychiatry* 34(suppl):164–169.

Power P (1999) Suicide and early psychosis. In: McGorry PD, Jackson HJ, eds, *Recognition and Management of Early Psychosis: A Preventive Approach.* New York: Cambridge University Press; 338–362.

Power P, McGorry PD (1999) Initial assessment of first-episode psychosis. In: McGorry PD, Jackson HJ, eds, *Recognition and Management of Early Psychosis: A Preventive Approach.* New York: Cambridge University Press; 155–183.

Power P, Elkins K, Adlard S et al (1998) Analysis of the initial treatment phase in first-episode psychosis. *Br J Psychiatr* 172(suppl.):71–76.

Power P, Bell R, Mills R et al (in press). Suicide prevention in first episode psychosis. The development of a randomized controlled trial of cognitive therapy for suicidal patients with early psychosis. *Aust NZJ Psychiatry.*

Rabinowitz J, Bromet EJ, Lavelle G et al (1998) Prevalence and severity of substance use disorder and onset of psychosis in first-admission psychotic patients. *Psychol Med* 28:1411–1419.

Rahman A, Mubbashar M, Harrington R, Gater R (2000) Annotation: developing child mental health services in developing countries. *J Child Psychol Psychiatr* 41:539–546.

Rapoport J, Giedd J, Blumenthal J et al (1999) Progressive cortical change during adolescence in childhood-onset schizophrenia. *Arch Gen Psychiatry* 56:649–654.

Regier DA, Kaelber CT, Rae DS et al (1998) Limitations of diagnostic criteria and assessment instruments for mental disorders. *Arch Gen Psychiatry* 55:109–115.

Remington G, Kapur S, Zipursky RB (1998) Pharmacotherapy of first-episode schizophrenia. *Br J Psychiatry* 172(suppl.):66–70.

Resch F, Parzer P, Brunner R, Koch E (in press) Early detection of psychosis and preventive strategies in adolescence. In: Brenner HD, Strik W, Genner R, eds, *Preventive Strategies in Schizophrenia.* Bern: Hogrefe and Huber.

Robinson D, Woerner MG, Alvir JM et al (1999a) Predictors of relapse following response from a first episode of schizophrenia or schizoaffective disorder. *Arch Gen Psychiatry* **56**:241–247.

Robinson D, Woerner MG, Alvir JM et al (1999b) Predictors of treatment response from a first episode of schizophrenia or schizoaffective disorder. *Am J Psychiatry* **156**:544–549.

Rosen A (2000) Ethics of early intervention in schizophrenia. *Aust NZ J Psychiatry* **34**(suppl): S208–S212.

Rosen A, Diamond RJ, Miller V, Stein LI (1997) Becoming real: from model programs to implemented services. In: Hollingsworth EJ, ed, *The Successful Diffusion of Innovative Program Approaches: New Directions for Mental Health Services*. San Franciso: Josey Bass; 27–41.

Rothschild AJ, Samson JA, Bessett MP, Carter-Campbell JT (1993) Efficacy of the combination of fluoxetine and perphenazine in the treatment of psychotic depression. *J Clin Psychiatry* **54**:338–342.

Schön DA (1990) *Educating the Reflective Practitioner: Toward a New Design for Teaching and Learning in the Professions*. San Francisco: Jossey-Bass.

Scott DL, Huskisson EC (1992) The course of rheumatoid arthritis. *Baillières Clin Rheumatol* **6**: 1–21.

Shafii M, Steltz-Lenarsky J, Derrick A et al (1988) Comorbidity of mental disorders in the post-mortem diagnosis of completed suicide in children and adolescents. *J Affect Disord* **15**:227–233.

Siris S, Bermanzohn P, Mason S, Shurwall M (1994) Maintenance imipramine therapy for secondary depression in schizophrenia. *Arch Gen Psychiatr* **51**:109–115.

Spencer E, Birchwood M, McGovern D (2001) Management of first-episode psychosis. *Adv Psychiatr Treat* **7**:133–140.

Spiker DG, Weiss JC, Dealy RS et al (1985) The pharmacological treatment of delusional depression. *Am J Psychiatry* **142**:430–435.

Spitzer RL (1998) Diagnosis and need for treatment are not the same. *Arch Gen Psychiatry* **55**:120.

Strakowski SM (1994) Diagnostic validity of schizophreniform disorder. *Am J Psychiatry* **151**: 815–824.

Strakowski SM, Keck PF Jr, McElroy SL et al (1995) Chronology of comorbid and principal syndromes in first-episode psychosis. *Compr Psychiatry* **36**:106–112.

Strakowski SM, McElroy SL, Keck PE, West S (1996) The effects of antecedent substance abuse on the development of first-episode psychotic mania. *J Psychiatr Res*, **30**:59–68.

Strakowski S, Keck P, McElroy S et al (1998) Twelve-month outcome after a first hospitalization for affective psychosis. *Arch Gen Psychiatry* **55**: 49–55.

Strauss JS, Hafez H, Liberman RP, Harding CM (1985) The course of psychiatric disorder, III: longitudinal principles. *Am J Psychiatry* **142**: 289–296.

Sullivan HS (1927, reprinted 1994) The onset of schizophrenia. *Am J Psychiatry* **151**:135–139.

Svedberg B, Mesterton A, Cullberg J (2001) First-episode, non-affective psychosis in a total urban population: a 5-year follow-up. *Soc Psychiatry Psychiatr Epidemiol* **36**:332–337.

Szymanski SR, Cannon TD, Gallacher F et al (1996) Course of treatment response in first-episode and chronic schizophrenia. *Am J Psychiatry* **153**: 519–525.

Tansella M, Thornicroft G (1998) A conceptual framework for mental health services: the matrix model. *Psychol Med* **28**:503–508.

Thornicroft G, Tansella M (1999) *The Mental Health Matrix: A Manual to Improve Services*. Cambridge: Cambridge University Press.

Tobin M, Chen L (1999) Initiation of quality improvement activities in mental health services. *J Qual Clin Pract* **19**:111–116.

Tobin MJ, Hickie IB, Yeo FM, Chen L (1998) Discussing the impact of first onset psychosis programs on public sector health services. *Australas Psychiatry* **6**:181–183.

Tohen M, Stoll AL, Strakowski SM et al (1992) The McLean first-episode psychosis project: six-month recovery and recurrence outcome. *Schizophr Bull* **18**:273–282.

Van Os J, Hanssen M, Bijl R, Ravelli A (2000) Strauss (1969) revisited: a psychosis continuum in the general population? *Schizophr Res* **45**:11–20.

Vazquez-Barquero J, Cuest M, Castanedo S et al (1999) Cantabria first-episode schizophrenia study: three year follow-up. *Br J Psychiatry* **174**:141–149.

Victorian Department of Infrastructure (2000) *Victoria in Future: Data*. Melbourne: Victorian Department of Infrastructure.

Wasylenki DA, Goering PN (1995) The role of research in systems reform. *Can J Psychiatry* **40**:247–251.

Welch M, Garland G (2000) The safe way to early intervention: an account of the SAFE (Southern Area First Episode) Project. *Australas Psychiatry* **8**:243–248.

Whitehorn D, Lazier L, Kopala L (1998) Psychosocial rehabilitation early after the onset of psychosis. *Psychiatr Serv* **49**:1135–1137,1147.

Wiersma D, Nienhuis FJ, Slooff CJ, Giel R (1998) Natural course of schizophrenic disorders: a 15-year\ followup of a Dutch incidence cohort. *Schizophr Bull* **24**:75–85.

Yung AR, McGorry PD (1996) The prodromal phase of first-episode psychosis: past and current conceptualizations. *Schizophr Bull* **22**:353–370.

Yung AR, McGorry PD, McFarlane CA, Patton G (1995) The PACE Clinic: development of a clinical service for young people at high risk of psychosis. *Australas Psychiatry* **3**:345–349.

Yung AR, McGorry PD, McFarlane CR et al (1996) Monitoring and care of young people at incipient risk of psychosis. *Schizophr Bull* **22**:283–303.

Yung A, Phillips L, McGorry P et al (1998a) Prediction of psychosis. *Br J Psychiatry* **172** (suppl 33):14–20.

Yung AR, Phillips LJ, McGorry PD et al (1998b) Can we predict first-episode psychosis in a high-risk group? *Int J Psychopharmacol* **13**:23–30.

Yung AR, Phillips LJ, Drew LT (1999) Promoting access to care in early psychosis. In: McGorry PD, Jackson HJ, eds, *Recognition and Management of Early Psychosis: A Preventive Approach*. New York: Cambridge University Press; 80–114.

Yung AR, Phillips LJ, Yven HP et al (in press) Psychosis prediction: 12-month follow-up of a high risk ('prodromal') group. *Schizophr Res*.

Ziguras SJ, Stuart GW (2000) A meta-analysis of the effectiveness of mental health case management over 20 years. *Psychiatr Serv* **51**:1410–1421.

Zipursky RB (2001) Optimal pharmacologic management of the first episode of schizophrenia. In: Zipurksy RB, Schulz SC, eds, *The Early Stages of Schizophrenia*. Washington, DC: American Psychiatric Publishing, Inc. 81–106.

Zipursky RB, Lambe EK, Kapur S, Mikulis DJ (1998) Cerebral gray-matter volume deficits in first episode psychosis. *Arch Gen Psychiatry* **55**:540–546.

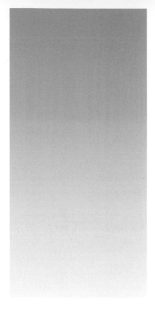

Index

Page numbers in **bold** refer to tables and those in *italics* to figures.